THE
EVERYTHING®
LOW CHOLESTEROL
BOOK
2ND EDITION

Dear Reader,

The first time I ever checked my cholesterol was my first week of medical school when we had to draw each other's blood. My cholesterol was awful! Up until that day, I had felt I could live however I wanted and it would never catch up to me. Over the following years, I saw the devastation caused by heart attacks and strokes and how cholesterol contributed to these disabling and deadly diseases. I did not want that to be my fate or the fate of those I cared about.

I have spent years studying and performing research on cardiovascular disease and cholesterol. Wanting to reduce my chances of early disease and disability, I have tried and implemented significant lifestyle changes. Through years of study and practice, I have learned what works and the challenges of making it work in our daily lives. In other words, I do not just talk the talk.

Now, as an emergency physician, I often see patients when it is too late. The greatest treatment for heart attacks, strokes, and other cardiovascular diseases is prevention. Hopefully, if you follow the advice and recipes in this guide, I won't see you in my emergency room.

Murdoc Khaleghi, MD

Welcome to the EVERYTHING® Series!

These handy, accessible books give you all you need to tackle a difficult project, gain a new hobby, comprehend a fascinating topic, prepare for an exam, or even brush up on something you learned back in school but have since forgotten.

You can choose to read an *Everything®* book from cover to cover or just pick out the information you want from our four useful boxes: e-questions, e-facts, e-alerts, and e-ssentials.

We give you everything you need to know on the subject, but throw in a lot of fun stuff along the way, too.

We now have more than 400 *Everything®* books in print, spanning such wide-ranging categories as weddings, pregnancy, cooking, music instruction, foreign language, crafts, pets, New Age, and so much more. When you're done reading them all, you can finally say you know *Everything®*!

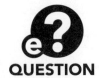

QUESTION

Answers to
common questions

FACT

Important snippets
of information

ALERT

Urgent
warnings

ESSENTIAL

Quick
handy tips

PUBLISHER Karen Cooper

DIRECTOR OF ACQUISITIONS AND INNOVATION Paula Munier

MANAGING EDITOR, EVERYTHING® SERIES Lisa Laing

COPY CHIEF Casey Ebert

ASSISTANT PRODUCTION EDITOR Jacob Erickson

ACQUISITIONS EDITOR Katrina Schroeder

ASSOCIATE DEVELOPMENT EDITOR Hillary Thompson

EDITORIAL ASSISTANT Ross Weisman

EVERYTHING® SERIES COVER DESIGNER Erin Alexander

LAYOUT DESIGNERS Colleen Cunningham, Michelle Roy Kelly, Elisabeth Lariviere, Ashley Vierra, Denise Wallace

Visit the entire Everything® series at *www.everything.com*

THE EVERYTHING®

LOW CHOLESTEROL BOOK
2ND EDITION

All you need to control your cholesterol and live a longer, healthier life

Murdoc Khaleghi, MD

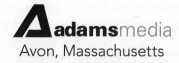

Avon, Massachusetts

This book is dedicated to all my patients who
taught me long before I could teach anyone.

An Everything® Series Book.
Everything® and everything.com® are registered trademarks of F+W Media, Inc.

Published by Adams Media, a division of F+W Media, Inc.
57 Littlefield Street, Avon, MA 02322 U.S.A.
www.adamsmedia.com

Contains material adapted and abridged from *The Everything® Low Cholesterol Cookbook* by Linda
Larsen, copyright © 2008 by F+W Media, Inc., ISBN 10: 1-59869-401-4, ISBN 13: 978-1-59869-401-7.

ISBN 10: 1-4405-0551-9
ISBN 13: 978-1-4405-0551-5
eISBN 10: 1-4405-0552-7
eISBN 13: 978-1-4405-0552-2

Printed in the United States of America.

10 9 8 7 6 5 4

Library of Congress Cataloging-in-Publication Data
Khaleghi, Murdoc.
The everything low cholesterol book / Murdoc Khaleghi. — 2nd ed.
p. cm. — (An everything series book)
Includes index.
ISBN 978-1-4405-0551-5
1. Hypercholesteremia—Prevention—Popular works. 2. Cholesterol—Health aspects—
Popular works. 3. Low-cholesterol diet—Popular works. I. Larsen, Linda Johnson. Everything
low-cholesterol cookbook. II. Title.
RC632.H83K43   2010
616.3'997—dc22   2010038814

This publication is designed to provide accurate and authoritative information with regard to the subject matter covered. It is sold with the understanding that the publisher is not engaged in rendering legal, accounting, or other professional advice. If legal advice or other expert assistance is required, the services of a competent professional person should be sought.

—From a *Declaration of Principles* jointly adopted by a Committee of the
American Bar Association and a Committee of Publishers and Associations

Many of the designations used by manufacturers and sellers to distinguish their products are claimed as trademarks. Where those designations appear in this book and Adams Media was aware of a trademark claim, the designations have been printed with initial capital letters.

This book is available at quantity discounts for bulk purchases.
For information, please call 1-800-289-0963.

Contents

Acknowledgments

I want to thank my literary agent, Neil Salkind at Studio B, and my acquisitions editor, Katrina Schroeder at Adams Media, for helping me help others. Thanks to Robert Kaplan and Luke Haseler for giving me my initial physiology, cardiovascular disease, and cholesterol research opportunities when I was younger. My research and studies also would not have been possible without the generous assistance and opportunities of the University of California, San Diego College and School of Medicine, and numerous scholarships and fellowships.

Thank you to Andy, Alyssa, and PJ, who have been incredibly patient with all my projects, letting me have time to both focus on them and sleep in between. Finally, thank you to Laura, the one person who could convince me to take a break from this book, at least once in a while.

The Top 10 Things You Need to Know about Your Cholesterol Levels

1. High cholesterol can increase your risk of heart attack, stroke, and other cardiovascular diseases.

2. Anyone can have high cholesterol.

3. There is no way to know if your cholesterol is high without getting it checked.

4. High total cholesterol matters far less than the type of cholesterol that is high.

5. For many cardiovascular diseases, the most effective treatment is prevention. Improving your cholesterol levels can reduce the chances of developing cardiovascular disease.

6. No matter your background, you can significantly change your cholesterol levels and reduce your chances of early death and disability.

7. Being active at least thirty minutes several times per week, not smoking, and reducing stress can significantly improve your cholesterol levels.

8. Eating fewer calories, saturated fats, and trans fats and consuming more complex carbohydrates, fiber, and unsaturated fats greatly benefits cholesterol levels.

9. Lifestyle changes are generally as or more effective at improving your cholesterol levels than medications.

10. The lifestyle changes that help your cholesterol also modify other contributors to cardiovascular disease, such as high blood pressure, high blood sugar, and obesity. Therefore, changing your lifestyle can save your life.

Introduction

YOU MAY HAVE HEARD of cholesterol. You may have even heard that it is bad. Every day it seems a new article comes out about what cholesterol does or what affects cholesterol. Not many people, though, know the full story.

Cholesterol over the years has earned a bad reputation. This reputation comes from cholesterol being known for decades to be a significant contributor to heart attacks, strokes, and other cardiovascular diseases. When people develop these debilitating and deadly diseases at a young age, cholesterol is often a factor. By understanding and managing cholesterol, you can avoid premature death and disability.

Cholesterol in excess builds up in your arteries, the blood vessels that deliver oxygen and nutrients to your brain. When these arteries get too clogged, parts of your organs cannot receive what cells need to survive. If this happened in the blood vessels to your brain, you would suffer a stroke, or in the blood vessels to your heart, a heart attack. These diseases can leave you disabled, paralyzed, or even kill you.

What you might not know is that you can recruit cholesterol to be on your side. There are different types of cholesterol; some clog arteries, but others clean up arteries. If you know how to lower the bad type and increase the good type, you can significantly prevent clogging or even unclog your arteries, reducing your chance of suffering heart attacks and strokes.

To start to manage your cholesterol, you need to get tested beginning at a fairly young age. These tests require repeating every few years, and if you are higher-risk, you may need testing more often to determine the proper treatment. This knowledge will help to guide you as you implement changes in your life to improve your cholesterol.

Cholesterol can be greatly influenced by your diet, physical activity, whether or not you smoke, your weight, and your levels of stress. By making certain changes in these areas, you can reduce your chance of early death and disability. Simple changes, such as eating fewer calories and bad fats in exchange for more fiber, nutrients, and good fats, can tremendously influence your cholesterol levels. Even a modest amount of physical activity a few days a week, no matter what the activity, can have a huge impact. Not smoking and reducing stress can reduce your bad cholesterol and raise your good cholesterol.

The changes that help your cholesterol can also reduce your risk for cardiovascular disease, as well as lower your blood pressure, weight, and blood sugar risks. Also, such changes in your lifestyle will give you more energy and an improved mood, improving the quality of your life.

Over the past twenty years, significant progress has been made in developing medications that improve cholesterol levels and reduce the chance of cardiovascular disease. These medications can create negative side effects, but the benefits may outweigh the risks.

Overall, by understanding cholesterol, how it acts, what you can do to manage it, and how to implement those actions, you can influence your future health tremendously, while potentially improving your current life.

CHAPTER 1

What Is Cholesterol?

You don't need to be a scientist to understand what cholesterol is and how to effectively manage your cholesterol levels for better health. You just need to care about your health. Take a moment to consider what is happening on the inside of your body to keep you alive. While most people take for granted that they don't need to think about the constant maintenance of their bodies, there are millions of processes working constantly to sustain their lives. Cholesterol is an essential part of this life process. Cholesterol keeps you going but can also stop you dead in your tracks. The better you understand cholesterol, the better you can choose which of these results will occur.

This Little Molecule

Cholesterol is a necessary and natural part of each and every cell in the human body and in the bodies of other animals. Cholesterol helps to maintain the structure of the walls of cells and works to keep brains healthy. The liver uses cholesterol as raw material to create important hormones such as adrenalin and sex hormones and to manufacture digestive enzymes such as bile acids that break down fats. Cholesterol is integral to thinking and sexual activity as well as innumerable other bodily functions.

FACT

Most gallstones that are formed in the gallbladder are composed primarily of cholesterol. The liver responds to the presence of dietary fat by producing cholesterol to synthesize bile to digest the fats. If you eat too much fat, the liver may overproduce cholesterol, leading to the formation of gallstones.

A healthy liver makes cholesterol, a waxy "lipid," or fatlike substance. In addition, you also acquire cholesterol from the food you eat. The big picture, however, is not quite so simple. Many other factors influence your cholesterol levels. Even if you are a vegetarian and don't eat foods that contain cholesterol, you will still have plenty of cholesterol in your body. Depending on the type of cholesterol and how much of each type, this can be a good or a bad thing.

Factors Affecting Cholesterol

Total cholesterol is the sum total of all the cholesterol in your bloodstream at a given time. There are different types of cholesterol, such as high-density lipoproteins (HDLs) and low-density lipoproteins (LDLs), which make up the total amount. Density refers to the weight of the lipoprotein. If cholesterol is HDL that means it is very compact, while if it is LDL that means it is less compact and more loose. In general, HDL is good cholesterol and LDL is bad cholesterol.

Several factors affect the total cholesterol levels in your bloodstream. These factors include the following:

- **What you eat:** Foods that come from animals, such as meats and eggs, contain cholesterol that you then absorb as well as saturated fats, which can convert into cholesterol in your body. Trans fats, contained in processed foods, are also converted into cholesterol.
- **Whether you are overweight:** Generally, the more fat you have, the more cholesterol you have. Therefore, weight loss can often lead to cholesterol loss.
- **Whether you smoke:** Smoking both raises your cholesterol and makes the cholesterol you have more harmful.
- **Whether you consume alcohol:** For years, scientists have noticed that moderate amounts of alcohol consumption can actually help your cholesterol levels. This comes with caution, as alcohol can worsen many other aspects of your health.
- **Whether you are inactive or active regularly:** People who are physically active on a regular basis have not only better levels of cholesterol, but they have more of the type that helps the body.
- **Whether you effectively manage stress in your life:** Research studies show that mental and emotional stress can raise your cholesterol and make the cholesterol you have more harmful to the body.
- **Your genes:** Your genes influence all your traits, including your cholesterol. If your parents had high cholesterol, you are more likely to have high cholesterol. In fact, there are certain common genetic disorders that will give you extremely high cholesterol, which can be incredibly harmful.
- **Your gender:** Before menopause, women have a natural advantage over men as female hormones help to maintain better cholesterol levels.
- **Age:** With time, cholesterol levels tend to worsen, causing cumulative harm which after years can be life-threatening.
- **What type of medications you take:** For certain individuals, medications can help to effectively manage cholesterol levels, while other medications can actually make cholesterol worse.

All of these will be discussed in detail throughout this book, with a focus on what you can do to improve your cholesterol levels. You may not be able to change your age, gender, or genes, but you can certainly change how you eat, whether you smoke, and how much you exercise.

A Complicated Puzzle

According to the National Cholesterol Education Program (NCEP), an authority on cholesterol recommendations, and guidelines issued by the federal government and supported by leading researchers and the American Heart Association (AHA), desirable total cholesterol results should be lower than 200mg/dL. Levels from 200 to 239mg/dL are considered borderline high. Total cholesterol levels of 240mg/dL and above are considered high.

Your total cholesterol levels, however, do not paint a complete picture of the health of your arteries. Because not all cholesterol is bad, you need to find out what type of cholesterol you have. Remember that cholesterol is essential to the health of every cell in your body and to the production of your hormones. Good cholesterol, or HDL, actually helps the body function well. To fully understand the health of your arteries and what is flowing in your bloodstream, you also need to find out about the levels of other blood fats, known as triglycerides.

Half the people whose total cholesterol levels come within the "desirable" levels have heart disease, so simply achieving this target does not guarantee that you are not at risk of heart disease. To truly evaluate your risk, you need to take into account all of the risk factors that apply to you. Pay particular attention if you have a family history of heart disease. Regardless of cholesterol levels, it is a good idea for everyone to observe healthy lifestyle habits, not only to lengthen your life but also to increase the quality of those additional years. Anyone can improve his or her health and reduce the risk of serious disease by improving his or her cholesterol.

FACT

Lipid is the chemical family name for fat. Its root is the Greek word *lipos,* meaning "fat." A blood lipid is a fat that circulates in the bloodstream. Cholesterol and triglycerides are both classified as blood lipids. A lipoprotein is a combination of fat surrounded and protected by protein to enable the fat to circulate within your mostly water-filled blood.

Why Cholesterol Is Good

The major players in the cholesterol picture are the liver and the blood fats. To help the body function, the liver takes cholesterol and fat from the blood to make new cholesterol. The liver manufactures both good and bad cholesterol, manages their release into the bloodstream, and collects cholesterol back from the bloodstream.

The body uses cholesterol and fat to build cell membranes, create essential hormones, and to form digestive enzymes. Fat and cholesterol need to be transported throughout the body. However, fat and cholesterol are oily, and blood is watery; oil and water do not mix. This makes fat and cholesterol difficult to transport on their own. The liver resolves this transport issue by combining and coating the cholesterol with substances that are fat on one side, touching the fat and cholesterol, and protein on the other side, touching watery blood. These are called lipoproteins, or combinations of fat and protein. The lipoprotein coating enables fat and cholesterol to travel in the bloodstream by shielding water-fearing fat with water-loving protein. The various types of lipoproteins are outlined in the following chart.

▼ **TYPES OF LIPOPROTEINS**

Name	Type of Lipoprotein	Nickname
HDL	High-density lipoprotein	"Good" cholesterol
LDL	Low-density lipoprotein	"Bad" cholesterol
VLDL	Very low-density lipoprotein	—
SDLDL	Small, dense, low-density lipoprotein	—
Lp(a)	Apolipoprotein (a) plus low-density lipoprotein	"Ugly" cholesterol

The Liver: Cholesterol Manufacturing Plant

Imagine a pickup and delivery service to and from the liver, which is the cholesterol manufacturing plant. Imagine that the lipoproteins are like delivery trucks that carry packages of cholesterol in the bloodstream. The function of the LDL delivery trucks is to package cholesterol and transport it out through the bloodstream to your various organs. Contrastingly, the function of the HDL "delivery trucks" is to pick up excess cholesterol "packages" from the bloodstream and return them to the liver for repackaging as needed.

In a healthy body, this efficient manufacturing, pickup, and delivery system maintains perfect balance. The LDLs go out to perform their functions at the receptor stops. HDLs pick up excess LDLs that the cells don't need and deliver them back to the liver for repackaging. Trucks circulate constantly, at all hours of the day and night, providing energy for quick fuel and for minimal storage reserves. The liver manufacturing plant naturally manages the entire process.

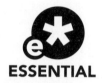

ESSENTIAL

The primary functions of the liver include metabolizing carbohydrates, proteins, and fats; storing and activating vitamins and minerals; forming and excreting bile to digest fats; converting ammonia to urea for elimination; metabolizing steroids; and acting as a filter by removing bacteria from blood. The liver also detoxifies substances such as drugs and alcohol.

When Good Cholesterol Turns Bad

Modern living conditions, however, overload and strain the system. By eating too much and moving too little, people make it all too easy for this delicately balanced delivery, pickup, and storage system to break down. The efficiency begins to fail when more LDL packages are transported in the bloodstream than are needed by the body's tissues. This excess LDL cholesterol continues to circulate in the bloodstream, increasing fat levels in the bloodstream and contributing to congestion in your arteries, the roadways where everything is transported.

If this excess LDL occurs at the same time that too few HDL trucks are available to collect and deliver it back to the liver for recycling, then the LDL cholesterol starts to collect on the arterial walls. Over time, this collection of debris on the arterial walls leads to a complete blockage, which then prevents blood flow that delivers essential oxygen for survival to the body's tissues. The body's tissues begin to die. If this happens in the muscle tissues of the heart, the result is a heart attack. If this happens in the brain, it causes a stroke. Almost any artery can get blocked, killing almost any area of your body, but the most common and important areas are your brain and heart.

The leading causes of the system breakdown are the following:

1. **Overproduction of LDL packages.** The liver produces too much LDL cholesterol for the body's needs and much more than the HDLs can pick up.
2. **Reduction of HDL pickup trucks.** The liver does not produce or release enough HDLs into the bloodstream to pick up the excess LDLs.
3. **Breakdown of liver management dispatch system.** The liver does not correctly signal to the body that it needs to pick up more LDLs.
4. **Damage to roadways.** Inflammation is present in the interior walls of the arteries.
5. **Transformation of LDL packages into litter.** Free radicals, which are breakdown products of some bodily functions, attach to certain LDL packages and "oxidize" them, causing them to become large and sticky and attach to blood vessel walls.

Scientists worldwide continue to conduct research so they can thoroughly understand the roles of the different types of lipoproteins and blood fats in the mechanisms behind heart disease. Evidence from research suggests that there are many LDL and HDL subtypes. Some of these subtypes are more harmful and others are more beneficial to health. For LDL cholesterol, particle size plays a significant role in the risk picture. People with higher numbers of the small, dense LDL particles, rather than the large, fluffy LDL particles, have a significantly higher risk of heart attack.

The Endothelial Lining

The endothelium, or endothelial lining, is the tissue that lines the inside of your blood vessels, through which nutrients travel through your bloodstream. Evidence from research studies shows that when this inner lining of the vessel walls becomes inflamed, so begins the formation of the clogging cholesterol plaque. White blood cells, which fight infection, go to the inflamed area, dragging with them other substances including calcium, cholesterol, and fats. Scientists have researched how to maintain the health of the endothelial lining to prevent the initial formation of plaque.

What Is Plaque?

Plaque is composed of bad cholesterol and calcium from the bloodstream, as well as other cellular waste products that get caught in the fat deposits. As the plaque grows larger, it hardens due to the deposition of calcium. It has an outer layer of scar tissue that covers the calcium and fats as well as the white blood cells that responded to the damaged arterial wall within.

Eventually the buildup of plaque can decrease or block blood flow to the heart or to the brain, starving these organs of essential oxygen and causing chest pains, a heart attack, or a stroke. This plaque buildup is known as atherosclerosis and is one of the most common types of heart disease. Plaque can begin to accumulate in childhood and develops so slowly in your body that its presence often grows without any signs to make you aware of it.

FACT

Often, heart disease is thought of as a killer in men, but it is also the number-one killer of women in America. Heart diseases kill more than half a million women each year—approximately one death per minute. The American Heart Association reports that heart disease claims more women's lives than the next seven causes of death combined!

Cholesterol's "High" Points

High-density lipoprotein (HDL) cholesterol, the pickup-truck fleet, is known as the "good" cholesterol. This is the compact, or high-density, form of cholesterol. When you understand how the liver's manufacturing and transport system works, it's easy to see why the HDLs are considered good—because HDLs help transport the excess LDL cholesterol from your arteries to the liver where it can be metabolized. That is why HDL is called the "good" cholesterol. For a healthy heart and circulatory system, you should have HDL cholesterol levels higher than 40mg/dL. The higher the level of your HDLs, the better it is for your health. People who have low levels of HDL cholesterol are at higher risk for heart disease.

According to the NCEP guidelines, an HDL level of 60mg/dL is considered a negative risk factor. A negative risk factor is like a bonus point that can decrease your heart attack or stroke risk. Since knowing the amount of your HDL cholesterol is an important aspect of assessing your overall risk of heart disease, it's a good idea to have your HDL cholesterol levels measured—not just your total cholesterol checked.

Cholesterol's "Low" Points

Low-density lipoprotein (LDL) cholesterol is known as the "bad" cholesterol; however, LDL cholesterol is bad for your body only if you have too much in your bloodstream or you have too much of the particularly harmful type. LDL cholesterol is an essential building block for cell membranes and the substance from which hormones, including cortisol and testosterone, are manufactured. The amount of LDL cholesterol that exceeds what your body needs, however, flows through your bloodstream and increases the likelihood of the formation of plaque that can block blood flow.

NCEP guidelines focus more on your types of cholesterol than your total cholesterol. For example, if you have high total cholesterol but it is mostly HDL, then that's a good thing! Unfortunately, most people's total cholesterol is composed mainly of LDL cholesterol, which is why having high cholesterol is generally considered bad for health.

Does the Total Really Matter?

A total cholesterol level includes different forms of cholesterol: LDL, the bad cholesterol that builds up in your arteries, and HDL, the good cholesterol that collects bad cholesterol from the blood vessels. If you have a lower level of LDL cholesterol and a higher level of HDL, you reduce the likelihood that you will have heart disease. One method to predict your risk of heart disease is to look at the ratio of total cholesterol to the level of HDL, or good cholesterol, at the time of your test. High levels of HDL in your bloodstream are good for your health. To calculate your ratio, divide your total cholesterol number by your HDL cholesterol. For men, a ratio of 4.5 to 1 or less is desirable. For women, the desired ratio is 4.0 to 1 or less.

ALERT

According to the American Heart Association, approximately 102 million Americans, or more than 50 percent of American adults, have total cholesterol levels of 200mg/dL or higher. This level indicates increased cardiovascular risk, and for most people, this total is composed mostly of LDL cholesterol. More than half of these Americans are unaware that they have high cholesterol.

Keep in mind, however, that this ratio is used as a rough predictor of risk, not to determine therapy. It is not enough simply to know total cholesterol and HDL levels—especially for planning treatment—as it does not provide a complete picture of the health of the circulatory system.

Triglycerides (TRGs)

Triglycerides, also referred to as TRGs, are a type of fat that circulates in your bloodstream. TRGs are composed of a sticky substance (called glycerol) and fatty acids. They can provide your body with a source of energy if needed. Triglyceride levels spike immediately after you eat and decrease slowly as the body processes nutrients from food that has been consumed. If muscles are working and active, triglycerides can provide needed fuel. If muscle cells do not use the circulating triglycerides to create energy, the TRGs are eventually deposited in the body's fat stores just like cholesterol, and just like cholesterol they can cause a clogging of your arteries.

People who are overweight, who drink alcohol excessively, who are diabetic, or who have other disorders are prone to having elevated triglyceride levels. Women tend to have higher triglyceride levels than men. Evidence from research shows that the risk of heart disease increases when the triglyceride level is too high, particularly when a person simultaneously has low levels of HDL cholesterol (fewer pickup trucks clearing these types of fats). Treatment is indicated for triglyceride levels above 150mg/dL.

Since eating affects all of your levels, you should fast for at least nine to twelve hours before you have a lipid profile test, which shows your HDL, LDL, triglycerides, and all other main types of fat and cholesterol. After you undertake this nine- to twelve-hour period without eating or drinking, the levels of these fats and cholesterols that are circulating in your bloodstream will more accurately reflect how much of these fats are consistently present in your blood, rather than what you recently ate.

▼ NCEP CHOLESTEROL AND TRIGLYCERIDE LEVEL GUIDELINES

Total Cholesterol Level	Category
Less than 180mg/dL	Optimal
Less than 200mg/dL	Desirable
200–239mg/dL	Borderline high
240mg/dL	High
LDL Cholesterol Level	LDL Cholesterol Category
Less than 100mg/dL	Optimal
100–129mg/dL	Near optimal/above optimal
130–159mg/dL	Borderline high
160–189mg/dL	High
190mg/dL and above	Very high
HDL Cholesterol Level	HDL Cholesterol Category
Less than 40mg/dL	Low
60mg/dL and above	High
Triglyceride Level	Triglyceride Category
Less than 150mg/dL	Normal
150–199mg/dL	Borderline high
200–499mg/dL	High
500mg/dL and above	Very high

Source: NIH Publication Nos. 01-3305 and 01-3290

Frequently Asked Questions

If I can't live without cholesterol, why is high cholesterol a problem?

Too much cholesterol in the blood can lead to blockage of the arteries. Fatlike deposits may build up inside arteries that provide blood to the legs, blood to the brain, or blood to the heart.

When blood flow through a coronary artery (blood to the heart) is completely blocked, an area of the heart muscle does not receive the blood and therefore the oxygen blood carries that the heart needs to survive. When this happens, a heart attack occurs. Plaque can also build up in the carotid arteries that supply blood to the brain. If this breaks free and a clot of it goes to the brain, it can cause a stroke. When plaque builds up in the blood vessels of the legs, it can cause leg pain, fatigue, cramping, or feelings of heaviness. This condition is known as peripheral arterial disease. When plaque builds up in the arteries that supply blood to the male sex organs, erectile dysfunction or impotence can result.

When I test my cholesterol, what information do I need to get?

The federal government guidelines recommend that every person who is age twenty or older should have a fasting lipoprotein profile at least once every five years. This test measures total cholesterol, LDL cholesterol, HDL cholesterol, and triglycerides. All of this information is relevant to get a picture of the health of your circulatory system.

FACT

People with very high cholesterol levels can reduce both their cholesterol and level of risk for a heart attack. According to the American Heart Association, drug therapy combined with lifestyle changes helps people with very high cholesterol reduce heart attacks by 34 percent and cardiac deaths by more than 40 percent.

What is the difference between good and bad cholesterol and triglycerides?

HDLs are known as the good type of cholesterol because their function is to gather excess LDL cholesterol in the body and return it to the liver. LDL cholesterol, although it serves a valuable purpose, is referred to as bad cholesterol because too much LDL cholesterol is harmful to the body. The reason excess LDL cholesterol is harmful is because it contributes to plaque formation on the inside of inflamed blood vessel walls.

Triglycerides are not similar to LDLs in terms of their function in the body, but they are similar in the way they cause harm to the body when present in excess. Like LDLs, triglycerides also travel through the bloodstream. Since triglycerides are a type of sticky blood fat, they also contribute to formation of plaque inside damaged blood vessel walls. Therefore, in general, most people want to increase HDL cholesterol levels and decrease LDL and triglyceride levels.

How can I increase my HDL cholesterol levels?

HDL cholesterol responds well to lifestyle changes. If you increase your physical activity each day or exercise regularly, it will stimulate the liver's production of HDLs. Losing excess weight can also improve your HDL profile. If you smoke cigarettes, you will increase your HDL levels simply by quitting your habit. If your HDLs are less than 35mg/dL, you may need drug therapy. Ask your health care provider what strategies are most suitable for you.

ALERT

Research has shown that identifying your cholesterol profile is far more important than knowing your total cholesterol. Levels of HDL and LDL provide an even more accurate assessment of the risk of coronary artery disease.

How does being more active help to lower cholesterol?

Regular physical activity can increase your HDL cholesterol, reduce LDL cholesterol, and reduce triglycerides. Since triglycerides are a blood fat, they are available to the body as a source of fuel for muscular activity. Therefore, people who are active can use up the triglycerides in their bloodstream as a source of energy.

Evidence from numerous research studies shows that moderate exercise, such as brisk walking, that adds up to a total of thirty minutes on most days of the week can improve your health. The great news is that you do not need to exercise vigorously or for hours at a time to achieve health benefits. In addition to burning up excess fats, moderate exercise also helps to reduce stress, which further enhances your well-being.

How does smoking affect cholesterol levels?

Cigarette smoke contains many toxic chemicals. These not only destroy lung tissue, they also contribute to plaque formation and adversely affect the nervous system, causing both heart rate and blood pressure to elevate. These chemicals contribute to reducing levels of good HDL cholesterol, raising LDL cholesterol, and accelerating the process of heart disease. While it is difficult to kick the smoking habit, the benefits of not smoking begin as soon as you quit.

If high cholesterol runs in my family, what, if anything, can I do to lower it?

Approximately 10 percent of American adults with high cholesterol are genetically predisposed to have this condition. If you have a family history of heart disease, it is even more important for you to work together with your health care provider to monitor your heart health with routine checkups annually.

Lifestyle factors such as physical activity, proper nutrition, not smoking, and effective stress management still matter. Even with a healthy lifestyle, your physician may still recommend drug therapy. With today's tools and knowledge, much can be done to manage the risks that you inherited. The information in this book is a great first step toward arming yourself with the necessary knowledge to empower yourself to positively manage your own health and well-being.

CHAPTER 2

Cholesterol and Heart Disease

In an instant, heart disease can tear a family apart. Abruptly, it can sever ties among spouses, parents and children, friends, neighbors, and other loved ones. Imagine how the sudden death or paralysis of you or a loved one would affect every aspect of your life. The good news in this grim scenario is that with knowledge and with action, you can take significant steps toward reducing the heavy toll from this disease. Understanding what heart disease is and how cholesterol contributes to it is an important first step.

What Is Heart Disease?

A healthy heart and well-functioning circulatory system are things that many people take for granted—that is, until one day they experience chest pains or breathlessness and realize that something in the body is no longer working the way it should. But what keeps a heart healthy? Or, what causes a heart to lose its ability to function properly?

The Structure and Function of the Heart

Before you can clearly understand what is going on when the heart does not work correctly, you should have a basic comprehension of its optimal structure and function. The human heart lies in the upper left center of the chest, next to the lungs. Blood flows into the right side of the heart and out of the left side. To guide the flow of blood in one constant direction, each chamber connects to the next one through valves that open when the heart contracts.

FACT

The circulatory system includes the heart, lungs, and all of the blood vessels. In the average person, these vessels would be 100,000 miles long if laid end-to-end. The heart pumps blood through these vessels to deliver oxygen and nutrients throughout the body and to remove carbon dioxide and other cellular waste products.

Blood that no longer contains as much oxygen because the oxygen has been used by the organs enters the right side of the heart through a large vein called the vena cava. This deoxygenated blood flows into the right heart. From the right ventricle, the blood enters the pulmonary artery to reacquire oxygen in the lungs. The newly oxygen-rich blood leaves the lungs and flows back to the heart's left side. When this section contracts, blood then rushes into the aorta to repeat its journey around the body. When blood reaches all the organs, it releases oxygen for the body to use to make energy. Once the blood gives up this oxygen, it returns to the heart to go back to the lungs to again acquire oxygen, and so on. This circulatory process continues automatically for as long as you live, and your life is dependent on it.

An electrical stimulus regulates the heartbeat. In the right atrium, a specialized group of cells—known as the sinoatrial (SA) node, or the sinus node—triggers the electrical impulses that travel across the heart muscle and cause the chambers of the heart to contract and push the blood along its path. The rate of the electrical impulses is regulated, but it can vary depending on different chemical stimulators in the body. By self-regulation of the rate of this firing, a healthy heart can respond to different needs as required by the demands of life.

For example, when you are reclining on a couch in a primarily horizontal position, your heart does not have to work as hard to circulate blood around your body since it does not have to flow against gravity. When you stand up from the couch—let's say to get a drink from the refrigerator—your heart must work harder to pump blood against gravity and to your working muscles. If you choose to play a sport or go for a run, often the heart has to work extra hard to meet the demands of your muscles that are quickly using oxygen. In a person with a healthy heart, all of these adaptations occur effortlessly. Many never pause to think about how their movements increase the demands on their circulatory system; they simply go and assume that their body will respond smoothly and easily.

The function of the heart and the circulatory system is to keep blood flowing continuously at a consistent rate. This ensures delivery of essential oxygen and nutrients to the body's tissues. Other processes that occur simultaneously through the circulation include the removal of waste products from cells back to the lungs, liver, and kidneys for filtering. A healthy nervous system is also important to a healthy circulatory system, since it affects heart rate and vessel function.

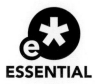

ESSENTIAL

A healthy heart is an electronically regulated muscular pump that is about the size of a fist. Each day and night, the average heart beats approximately 100,000 times and pumps 2,000 gallons of blood. Over a normal life span, the heart will beat more than 2.5 billion times.

What Can Go Wrong with the Heart?

Unfortunately, the heart doesn't always function perfectly. To comprehend the role of cholesterol, the process of atherosclerosis, and their impact on heart diseases, you need to be able to understand them in the context of the range of potential heart problems. There are several disorders that can have a negative effect on the circulatory process by reducing blood flow. Some of these disorders are genetic; others are either caused by or worsened by atherosclerosis that results from the presence of harmful types of cholesterol circulating in the bloodstream. The most common disorders are:

- Arrhythmias, or malfunctions of the electrical system, causing an irregular heartbeat
- Congestive heart failure, or weakness of the muscular pump, causing fluid to back up into the lungs and other organs
- Congenital defects, such as a hole between the two atrial chambers (an atrial septal defect)
- Narrowing of the heart valves from calcification (stenosis) or from tumors in the heart
- Valve leakage, known as insufficiency, keeping the blood from flowing through chambers optimally
- Damage to the heart muscle itself from blockage of coronary arteries due to atherosclerosis

Each of these disorders results in a heart muscle that is not capable of pumping blood sufficiently. All of these, with the exception of congenital defects, can be caused by heart attacks.

When and Why the Heart Stops Working

If cholesterol builds up in the blood vessels that feed oxygen to the heart, then the heart cells no longer receive oxygen and cannot function properly. The blood vessels that are clogged may feed the whole heart or only some of the heart. Depending on how much of the heart is starved for oxygen, symptoms may be unnoticeable or may quickly escalate to death. The heart may just stop pumping. If your heart stops pumping, every organ, from the brain to the kidneys, will stop working, which will result in death in a few minutes.

Alternatively, your heart may become very weak at pumping. When the heart cannot pump blood well, the fluid the heart is trying to pump backs up into the lungs, making it difficult to breathe. This difficulty can make even the slightest tasks, such as going up stairs, incredibly challenging. The heart may not fire in the rhythm it is supposed to. The heart may fire too fast, causing too much demand on the muscle. It could fire too slow, causing not enough blood and oxygen to pump out to the rest of the body. Or it could fire irregularly, causing blood clots to form. These blood clots could travel to other organs and may contribute to strokes or other organ failures.

The Process Can Be Fast or Slow

The clots that block blood flow to your heart may come on slowly or quickly. The slow process, called atherosclerosis, is the progressive buildup of plaque within blood vessels. Pathways become smaller and smaller, until not enough blood will flow through the vessel to meet the demand. The process is quick when plaque breaks in one blood vessel and travels to a smaller vessel where it is trapped and stops all blood flow. This is an embolism. The two processes can also work together, where atherosclerosis thins the vessel, and plaque gets stuck in the thinner vessel.

What Is a Stroke?

The brain needs oxygen to survive, like the heart and every other part of the body. It obtains that oxygen from blood that is transported through the blood vessels. Any obstruction to that blood flow will cause the brain to die. And just as every part of your body is dependent on the heart, so is every part of your body dependent on the brain. The brain controls all aspects of thinking, movement, and sensation, and if it stops working, everything else will, too. A stroke is essentially a "brain attack." Both atherosclerosis and embolisms may obstruct blood flow to the brain and cause the dysfunction of some parts or nearly all of the brain. Strokes are just as devastating to people and families as heart attacks, and in some ways can be even more devastating.

Strokes can cause permanent damage that affects every aspect of basic neurologic functioning. They can paralyze, making the victim unable to use a certain extremity or side of the body. They can affect thinking, so that the victim cannot speak with the right words. They can also affect understanding—many sufferers are not able to comprehend what is in front of them. Strokes can steal away the ability to remember the most basic things. They can even affect swallowing, forcing patients to eat through a tube inserted directly in the stomach. A severe stroke can result in extreme disability or death. According to the Centers for Disease Control and Prevention, when considered separately from other cardiovascular diseases, stroke is the third-leading cause of death in the United States.

ALERT

If you feel that someone may have suffered a stroke or heart attack, get the victim to a hospital as soon as possible. Be sure to call the hospital and let staff there know you are on the way or, even better, call 911 and await ambulance arrival.

Strokes are less treatable than heart attacks. While there are still certain treatments for strokes, they are far less expansive and effective than the multitude of heart attack treatments that have developed over the last decade. Unless the stroke is treated within several hours of onset, most of what doctors can do is just watchful waiting to see whether the stroke results in disability. Further tests and treatments are only potentially able to prevent future strokes. Even within the first few hours, the treatments are often ineffective. Since treatment options are minimal once someone has a stroke, the main method of combating strokes is trying to prevent them from ever occurring. Prevention is also the best way to fight heart attacks and other cardiovascular disease. Managing cholesterol has become a key aspect of that prevention.

A mild or mini-stroke, described as a transient ischemic attack (TIA), can end in a matter of minutes. The damage can include mild weakness or numbness in an arm or a leg or slight difficulty with speech. This can be a warning sign for a larger impending stroke.

According to the American Heart Association and American Stroke Association, approximately 40,000 more women than men have strokes annually. Experts believe that this is because women tend to live longer than men, and the highest rates for stroke are among those in the oldest age groups.

What Is Peripheral Arterial Disease?

Atherosclerosis not only affects the arteries that supply blood to the heart and to the brain, but it can also affect the vessels that supply blood to the legs. This condition is known as peripheral arterial disease (PAD). Clogging of these arteries leads to discomfort in the legs that can become more severe as time goes on. What is particularly worrisome is that you are much more likely to have a heart attack or stroke if you have this condition.

Warning signs and symptoms of PAD include:

- Cramping, heaviness, fatigue, or aching of the buttocks, thighs, or calves when walking
- Leg pain that occurs when you walk uphill, carry heavy loads, or walk quickly
- Aching of the foot that worsens at night and is relieved by standing up or by allowing the foot to hang off the edge of the bed
- Leg pain that stops when you stand still or rest

If allowed to progress, peripheral arterial disease can lead to lack of blood flow to the feet. The feet, like any other body part, cannot survive without blood flow. If not corrected in time, the only treatment is amputation.

Atherosclerosis and Erectile Dysfunction

Erectile dysfunction is often associated with atherosclerotic plaque buildup. Impotence can be an early warning sign of cardiovascular disease. According to the National Institute of Diabetes and Digestive and Kidney Diseases, about 5 percent of forty-year-old men and between 15 to 25 percent of sixty-five-year-old men experience erectile dysfunction. In addition, when smoking is part of the picture, the odds of erectile dysfunction increase even further. Male smokers have approximately a 30 percent higher risk for erectile dysfunction when compared with nonsmokers. However, just as hardening of the arteries is not inevitable with aging, neither is the loss of potency. Maintaining health of the heart and circulatory system can also help to maintain this aspect of youthful vigor and vitality.

Intestinal Atherosclerosis

Even the intestines' blood flow can become blocked, causing intense stomach pains. Sadly, this disease is incredibly hard to diagnose as there are so many other causes of stomach pain. By the time an intestinal stroke is discovered, death is the usual outcome. Once again, the best method of treating this disease is avoidance through prevention.

What's Cholesterol Got to Do with It?

As previously explained, the two biggest killers, strokes and heart disease, come in a variety of life-threatening forms. All these diseases are referred to as cardiovascular diseases (CVDs). CVDs also include high blood pressure, coronary heart disease, congestive heart failure, stroke, rheumatic heart disease, artery diseases, pulmonary heart disease, and congenital cardiovascular defects.

Atheroembolic disease of the arteries that supply the heart is known as coronary heart disease or coronary artery disease (CAD).

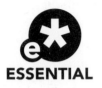

ESSENTIAL

According to government statistics, if all forms of major cardiovascular disease (CVD) were eliminated, life expectancy would rise by almost seven years. Compared with that, if all forms of cancer were eliminated, the gain would be only three years. The probability at birth of eventually dying from major CVD is almost 50 percent, while the chance of dying from cancer is approximately 22 percent.

It is possible for a person to have more than one type of cardiovascular disease at the same time. In fact, many people have multiple cardiovascular disorders at once, as having one cardiovascular disorder increases the risk for having another. For example, a person may have both coronary artery disease and high blood pressure. Coronary artery disease is responsible for more than half of all heart attacks in men and women under age seventy-five.

Scientists now know that atherosclerosis can start in childhood. Researchers have found the beginning of fatty streaks in the arteries of children as young as three years old. The average American has significant buildup in his arterial walls by middle age. In women, possibly because of the protective effects of estrogen, the thicker buildups do not begin to show up until after menopause.

Even without the impact of a stroke or heart attack, atherosclerosis advances the aging process. Healthy circulation in the body is the source of nutrition and life for the cells. As this circulation is slowly cut off, it impairs the functioning of your cells. Atherosclerosis does not need to be inevitable. With knowledge of the mechanisms that contribute to this disease, you can take steps to reduce your risks and to prolong your youthful vitality and energy.

Atherosclerosis and Coronary Artery Disease

The principal cause of coronary artery disease is atherosclerosis, or hardening of the arteries. *Atherosclerosis* comes from the root words *atheroma* and *sclerosis*, which means "to harden." As you have learned, atherosclerosis is a process that leads to a group of diseases characterized by the thickening of artery walls. The thickening results from a buildup of plaque on the arterial walls, with this plaque growth being highly dependent on your HDL and LDL cholesterol levels. Plaque is made up of various types of debris including triglycerides that collect on areas of inflammation on blood vessel walls, causing more and more narrowing of the passage through which blood can flow. (See Chapter 1 for more information on plaque buildup.)

Plaque is formed in a variety of shapes and sizes. Small plaques accumulate throughout the arteries in the entire body and can be difficult to detect. Doctors can more easily discover the large, hardened plaques in the coronary arteries.

ALERT

According to the National Heart, Lung, and Blood Institute, heart attack risk for both men and women is highest when a person has a combination of low HDL levels and high LDL levels. People with low levels of HDL are also at a high risk regardless of the level of their total cholesterol.

Small plaque buildups, however, are just as concerning as thick, hard plaques. Researchers have determined that these smaller plaques are less solid on the outside and, consequently, less stable. These small, unstable plaques are much more likely to rupture and release the cholesterol mass into the bloodstream. This concentrated cholesterol contributes to formation of blood clots. If a small plaque buildup in the coronary arteries ruptures and forms a blood clot, it can trigger a heart attack.

Many factors determine the number, size, and nature of these plaques, but one of the most important of those factors is your cholesterol. Specifically, the amount of LDL cholesterol and triglycerides you have depositing in these plaques and the amount of HDL cholesterol you have taking cholesterol away from these plaques are significant determinants of their severity.

Remember, most people with cardiovascular disease will not get a warning. Most people will not have advance notice that reveals deadly plaques before they happen. To avoid the two most common and deadliest diseases in society, you must act even before the warning signs, because often by the time you get warning signs, it may be too late. By understanding the nature of LDL and HDL cholesterol, only then can you act to prevent early death or disability.

You Have the Power to Improve Your Health

There are many things about yourself that you cannot change. You cannot change your age. You cannot change your genes. You cannot change what you have once done to your body, whether you used to smoke or eat poorly. Now, though, whether you are young or old, male or female, you can improve your health and reduce your risk of cardiovascular diseases by consistently monitoring and managing your cholesterol levels. You can make lifestyle changes that significantly lower risks of cardiovascular disease, regardless of your genetic heritage. Even if you already have coronary artery disease, you can reap benefits. In fact, being higher risk for a cardiovascular event can mean even greater benefits than those who are lower-risk by managing your cholesterol levels through greater risk reduction. Research evidence shows that decreasing your blood-cholesterol levels can slow, stop, and even reverse plaque buildup over time. As you lower your LDL cholesterol levels and increase your HDL levels, you can reduce the cholesterol content in the unstable plaque that has built up in the arterial walls. You can get your HDL trucks to start transporting plaque material back to your liver for metabolism, rather than let LDL sit and continue to grow in your arteries. Accordingly, you will reduce your future risks of having a heart attack or stroke.

Through effective cholesterol management, you can cut your risks of having a future heart attack and add valuable years to your life. At the same time, beyond extending your longevity, improving your lifestyle habits can also enrich the quality of those additional years of living. It is possible to become even healthier as you age; suffering years of disease, disability, and loss of vitality is not anyone's necessary fate. Adopting healthy habits extends your youthfulness and enhances your feelings of well-being. You can make a difference to improve your odds and to get even more enjoyment out of life.

Think: How hard do you work to earn money? Do you sometimes wish there were extra hours in the day? How much time and effort do you put into helping your loved ones? By working to improve your cholesterol levels, you can add years to your life. You can save thousands of dollars in medical bills and perhaps far more in productivity. You can make sure you maximize how much life you are able to give to your loved ones and minimize how much your loved ones will need to take care of you. The things you do to improve your cholesterol will help with your future health and will greatly improve the life you live now.

CHAPTER 3

It's Not All about Cholesterol

As with most things in life, you are not completely in control of whether you will develop heart disease. At the same time, however, you are far from being totally helpless. There are many steps you can take to lessen your risk of developing heart disease. But before you can reduce your risks and improve your odds, you need to know what those risks are. Most risks you can influence, some you cannot. The more risk factors you have, the more important it is to try to reduce those risk factors, including your cholesterol.

What Else Matters?

Heart disease is what is described as a multifactorial disease. This means that multiple factors contribute to the development and progression of the disease. One risky characteristic alone, such as your age, may be enough to trigger the disease. However, a combination of factors, such as age, inactivity, smoking, and improper nutrition, will put you at much higher risk for heart attacks and strokes. The more risk factors that you possess, the greater your likelihood of having the disease. Fewer risk factors, on the other hand, mean less likelihood of having the disease.

Identifying Risk Factors

After many years of research, scientists have identified risk factors for heart disease. Investigators conducted a landmark long-term study observing over 4,000 male and female residents of Framingham, Massachusetts. This study is world-renowned for the size of its database and has been the landmark study used for decades. Researchers measured blood pressure, recorded cholesterol levels, and noted connections between the data and the participants who suffered from heart disease over the term of the study. This is not only one of the largest studies ever done, but it is also one that emphasized the paramount importance of cholesterol.

A clear relationship emerged between those who had heart attacks and those who also had high blood-cholesterol levels. Other causal factors also emerged. The sum total of evidence from this and other studies provides researchers with the ability to assess risk by analyzing the presence or absence of these identifiable risk factors. Numerous studies since have verified the important link between cholesterol and your risk of cardiovascular disease.

FACT

To determine your risk score according to the information gathered by the Framingham Study, use the online calculator at *http://hp2010 .nhlbihin.net/atpiii/calculator.asp?usertype=prof*. Keep in mind that subjects in this study were primarily Caucasian, middle-aged, and without heart disease. It may not be completely accurate for other groups, but it is still useful as a general guide.

Any condition that indicates the presence of atherosclerosis indicates a high risk of coronary artery disease. In other words, having a stroke puts you at higher risk for a heart attack. The reverse is also true. Researchers today also identify diabetes as a condition that creates a high risk of coronary artery disease. Diabetes is classified as carrying the equivalent risk of any of the other diseases that indicate the presence of heart disease.

Keep in mind that the basis for these risk factors is data from large-population studies and is simply a reflection of profiles of those among the population who had a heart attack. Historically, however, research studies have not included in their database sufficient numbers of women, people from ethnic minorities, people from a variety of economic backgrounds, or people from a variety of lifestyles with different levels of access to health care. More recently, though, studies have started to incorporate these historically underrepresented groups. The studies have shown that cholesterol has an important role in determining these groups' risks for heart attacks and strokes.

The leading risk factors for heart disease are as follows:

- High LDL cholesterol
- Low HDL cholesterol
- Diabetes
- Cigarette smoking or inhaling secondary smoke
- Hypertension or high blood pressure
- Unmanaged stress
- Physical inactivity or a sedentary lifestyle
- Excess weight
- Family history of heart disease
- Age and gender

As you can see, this list includes several risk factors you can actively do something about. A few factors, such as your family history (or genetic predisposition) and your age and gender are things you cannot change or control. The good news, however, is that you can make a strong impact on your modifiable risk factors. The way you choose to live your life every day plays a very important role in reducing your risk of heart disease. What you do makes a difference.

Before taking action, it helps to understand why these factors create risk and how they increase your chances of having a heart attack. When you clearly see the relationship between your unhealthy habits and how they can cause your own death or disability, or the loss of a loved one, it is easy to get motivated to improve your lifestyle and the lifestyle of your family.

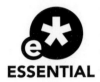

ESSENTIAL

It is well worth your time to assess where you stand today in terms of your risk for heart disease. With that information, you can get motivated either to keep up the great work or to make the changes that you need to lower your risks, as well as the risks of those whom you love. Don't wait to get started. Get going right away toward creating a healthy lifestyle.

Diabetes as a Risk Factor

Diabetes is a condition characterized by the failure of insulin to perform its normal functions. In a healthy body, the pancreas produces the hormone insulin and releases it into the bloodstream. The body uses this insulin to convert sugar, starches, and other foods into stored energy. When the system is not functioning normally, the bloodstream is overloaded with excess sugar. Scientists have not yet identified the exact cause of diabetes, but they believe that genetics, excess weight, and inactivity all contribute to development of the disease.

Evidence from numerous research studies shows that people with diabetes mellitus have as much risk of having a heart attack as those who are already diagnosed with heart disease. To put this risk into statistical terms, people with diabetes have a 15 to 20 percent chance of having a heart attack within a ten-year period. This is the same level of risk as a person who is diagnosed with coronary artery disease. Furthermore, a person with diabetes has twice the likelihood of dying from a heart attack than a person who does not have diabetes. Diabetes, like cholesterol and coronary artery disease, is a silent killer. You may not know you are diabetic for a long time, possibly until it is too late.

Because of the increased risk of heart disease associated with diabetes, the federal government guidelines recommend that people who are diabetic pursue the same cholesterol goals as those who have heart disease. Adults age forty-five and over should be tested to determine whether they are diabetic. See Chapter 14 for more information on diabetes and its relationship to heart disease.

ALERT

According to the American Diabetes Association, approximately 23 million Americans have diabetes. Health care professionals have diagnosed approximately two-thirds of these people. As many as one-third of the total people who have this condition, however, are not aware they have it.

The Metabolic Syndrome

Researchers have identified a cluster of symptoms including abdominal obesity, high triglycerides, low HDL levels, high blood pressure, and a high fasting blood-glucose level as contributors to a higher risk for heart disease. Studies have substantiated that individuals who have a cluster of three or more of these factors have a greater risk of heart disease than someone who may have only one or two of the risk factors, as one would expect.

This clustering of several risk factors is described as the "metabolic syndrome." The reason for this reference is that the metabolic syndrome focuses on risk factors that have a metabolic origin. Carrying excess weight and leading an inactive lifestyle increase the likelihood of developing the syndrome. Medical experts agree that when an individual has diabetes or has the cluster of factors that comprise the metabolic syndrome, she has a very high likelihood of having a heart attack. In addition to those conditions, there are several factors that can exacerbate the situation. See Chapter 14 for further information on the metabolic syndrome.

What You Cannot Change

Among the many risk factors, some you cannot influence, such as your genes or age. Some, on the other hand, you can have a powerful influence over. While it is important to recognize all your risk factors to determine your overall risk, it is more important to focus on those you can change. Focusing on these will have the most positive impact on your future. Equally important is knowing the best way to influence your risk factors. Treating one risk factor often affects other risk factors, thereby reducing your overall chances of developing cardiovascular disease.

Your Family History

Family history is an important consideration when determining your risk for heart disease. If you have a first-degree female relative (mother, sister, or daughter) under the age of sixty-five or a first-degree male relative (father, brother, son) under fifty-five who has heart disease, that is a risk factor for you. If your parents have had heart disease, then you are more likely to develop heart disease.

QUESTION

If my family has heart disease, what can I do to minimize risk?
Maintain healthy habits such as eating nutritious foods, keeping a healthy weight, staying active on a regular basis, and managing stress. Be sure to check your cholesterol levels and blood pressure regularly.

Of course, no one can change his genes, but if you have a family history of heart disease, it is even more important for you to assess your risk factors and to have annual checkups. While genetics are powerful, they do not have to determine your fate. Take control of the factors that you can change.

Your Age and Gender

Men are at a greater risk than women of developing heart disease in middle age. From the age of forty-five, a man's risk of heart disease increases, and this risk continues to increase with age. By the age of sixty-five, half of all American men are likely to have coronary artery disease.

Women enjoy some protection from heart disease that may come from the hormone estrogen. Women who are fifty-five years of age and older, however, are at an increased risk of heart disease. Hormone replacement therapy has not been shown to reduce this risk. As with men, this risk continues to increase with age. By the age of sixty-five, a third of all American women are likely to have coronary artery disease.

You can't change your age, but you can improve other health habits to create a more healthy and enjoyable life. By following healthy habits, you can not only extend your years of life, but you can also add vitality to those later years. People who observe healthy habits when younger also tend to have much less disease and disability in their later years of life.

What You Can Change

The risk factors you can change are far more numerous than those you cannot change, meaning you have a major influence over your risk for a heart attack and stroke. By learning what you can change and how you can change, you can prevent early disease and disability while adding energy and productivity to your life. You can save on medical bills and give time and energy to those around you.

Cigarette Smoking and Secondhand Smoke

Smoking is a risk factor because smokers have twice the risk of developing heart disease as nonsmokers in the same condition. Also, a smoker who has a heart attack is more likely to die from it than a nonsmoker. Cigarette smoking is the greatest risk factor for sudden cardiac deaths. Smoking low-tar or low-nicotine cigarettes does not make any difference in reducing your risk of heart disease. Nonsmokers who are frequently exposed to secondhand smoke also have an increased risk of developing heart disease.

Smoking contributes to heart disease because the chemicals that are inhaled from cigarette smoke reduce the amount of the good HDL cholesterol in your bloodstream. In addition, nicotine increases the rate of the heartbeat and constricts arteries, leading to higher levels of blood pressure and stress on the heart and circulatory system. Some researchers believe that this can also lead to damage to arterial walls, making them more susceptible to plaque formation. Carbon monoxide reduces the amount of oxygen available to your body by up to 15 percent. Not only does this starve the body's tissue of essential oxygen, it also reduces the amount of oxygen delivered to fuel the heart muscle.

If you change this negative habit and quit smoking, you immediately begin to reduce your risk of heart disease. You also reduce your risks for lung cancer, lung disease, and other types of cancer. Your friends and loved ones reap the benefits of having you no longer subject them to second-hand smoke. See Chapter 12 for further information on the harmful effects of smoking and how to quit.

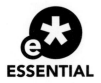

ESSENTIAL

Increasing evidence shows that secondhand smoke can break down antioxidant defenses, leading to damage to the endothelial lining of blood vessels, which represents the beginning of atherosclerosis. Studies show that oxidative stress is significantly higher in children exposed to secondhand smoke, increasing their later risk of heart disease, even if exposure consists of fewer than twenty cigarettes (one pack) per day by one parent.

High Blood Pressure

High blood pressure, also referred to as hypertension, is a risk factor for heart disease and stroke. Approximately one in every four American adults, or over 65 million people, has high blood pressure. If untreated, high blood pressure can compromise the functioning of the heart and the circulatory system.

High blood pressure occurs when the pressure of blood flowing through the blood vessels increases and remains elevated. This increase in pressure means that the blood flow is pushing against the arterial walls with a stronger-than-normal force. Over time, this increased pressure damages the arterial walls by causing them to become thicker and stiffer. The arterial walls lose elasticity and become more damaged. Research shows that damaged arterial walls are more likely to attract cholesterol and fats, which then form plaque. As you know, this plaque formation leads to blockage of the arteries that can cause a heart attack or stroke.

In addition to contributing to arterial damage and consequent plaque formation, prolonged high blood pressure forces the heart to work harder and enlarge. Over time, the heart fails to function normally and cannot fully pump out all the blood it receives. As after a heart attack, a weak heart can cause fluids to back up into the lungs and can rob the rest of the body of the blood supply that it needs. This condition is known as congestive heart failure. Also, the heart having to pump against more pressure increases the demands of the heart, increasing the need for oxygen. If the supply of oxygen does not meet the demand, such as when the blood vessels become constricted due to atheroembolic disease, you are at much higher risk for a heart attack.

FACT

Blood pressure is measured in millimeters of mercury (mmHg) and consists of two numbers usually written one over the other. The top number reflects the systolic blood pressure reading—this is a measure of the pressure when your heart contracts, pumping the blood out. The bottom number reflects diastolic blood pressure. This reading measures the pressure when your heart rests, refilling with blood in between contractions.

Ideally, your blood pressure should be lower than 140 mmHg over 90 mmHg (usually spoken as "140 over 90" and written as 140/90). If either your systolic, the higher number, or your diastolic blood pressure, the lower number, reading is higher than that, you may have high blood pressure. High blood pressure for a day, a week, or a month is not significantly harmful. Having high blood pressure for years, though, significantly increases your risk for cardiovascular disease.

If high blood pressure is treated, the risk of heart disease and stroke is reduced. Blood pressure can be managed by losing as little as five to ten pounds of extra weight, exercising regularly, reducing stress, and eating plenty of fruits, vegetables, and low- or nonfat dairy products.

Foods that can increase blood pressure for people who are sensitive to salt are processed meats, cheeses, canned foods like soups and vegetables, salty crackers and snack foods, salad dressings and condiments like soy sauce or barbecue sauce, and any other foods prepared with salty seasonings. Caffeine and alcoholic beverages can elevate blood pressure in some people. Foods that can reduce blood pressure levels are fruits and vegetables that are rich in potassium. This can include any type of dried fruit as well as bananas and melons.

High blood pressure is dangerous because it usually gives no warning signs or symptoms, like diabetes and high cholesterol. The only way to know whether your blood pressure is high is to get it checked, and not just once. Your blood pressure naturally changes during the day and rises dramatically when you are anxious. Some people simply become nervous when they are in the doctor's office, resulting in a higher reading. Drugstore machines typically are not as accurate as manual measurements. To determine whether you have high blood pressure, you will need to have it checked on several occasions and at different times of the day.

ALERT

According to the American Heart Association, of all the people with high blood pressure, less than half are on an adequate therapy. If you have high blood pressure, discuss all treatment options, including lifestyle changes and drug therapy, with your health care provider.

It is far better to keep your blood pressure from getting high in the first place. If you find that your blood pressure is not high, take steps to keep it that way. Keep your weight in a healthy range; aim to lose at least five to ten pounds if you are overweight; get more physically active; choose heart-healthy foods; and if you smoke, quit. All these lifestyle changes will help your cholesterol profile, as well.

Excess Weight

Those who carry excess weight are at an increased risk of heart disease, high blood pressure, stroke, and diabetes, among other things. Carrying excess weight increases the strain on the heart and circulatory system as well as on other body systems.

Just as the body needs a certain amount of LDL cholesterol to survive, it also needs a certain amount of body fat. However, excess body fat contributes to an increase in the natural production of higher levels of LDL cholesterol by the liver and to lower levels of HDL cholesterol. The delicate balance of the body's production and collection system of cholesterol becomes disturbed when the body carries additional fat stores. While the exact amount of fat that represents an excessive amount seems to vary from one individual to another, there seems to be a point at which too much body fat starts to harm, rather than to support, optimum health.

Conversely, when a person sheds excess body fat, the body's natural balancing mechanisms can begin to function effectively again. By losing excess fat, a person can stimulate the liver to decrease the production of LDL cholesterol and to increase the production of HDL cholesterol. This change can actually start to restore health to the circulatory system.

The answer to the question of what is a healthy weight, however, is not a simple one. A healthy weight varies from one individual to another. An individual's healthy weight range can depend on a number of factors, including age, gender, ethnicity, body type, and personal situation, such as whether he or she is an elite athlete or pregnant or lactating. An estimation of healthy weight is the body-mass index, or BMI. This is a calculation based on your height and weight to determine whether you are in your ideal weight range.

FACT

To calculate BMI, take your weight in kilograms and divide it by the square of your height in meters. You can use pounds and inches instead, multiplying your result by 703 to convert. You can also use the National Heart, Lung, and Blood Institute's BMI calculator at *www.nhl bisupport.com/bmi* to calculate your BMI, or see Appendix B.

If you are in the 18.5–24.9 range, you are considered to be at a healthy weight. If you are over 25, then you are considered overweight. The BMI is limited, as it does not factor body composition, which may be different for various people such as pregnant women or muscular athletes.

Lack of Physical Activity

Lack of exercise is an important risk factor that is largely within your control. People who are sedentary have twice the risk of heart disease compared with those who are active.

Researchers from the National Institute on Aging have said that if exercise were a prescription drug, it would be the most widely prescribed medication. Adding some form of an endurance activity into your daily life conditions your heart, lungs, circulatory system, muscles, bones, brain, and nervous system. Being physically active reduces your risk of heart disease, and it reduces your risk of high blood pressure, diabetes, cancer, back pain, cognitive disorders like Alzheimer's, and countless other diseases. Every day there seems to be a new study showing how exercise reduces the risk of a certain disease. Regular physical activity increases your levels of HDL (good cholesterol) and lowers your level of LDL (bad cholesterol). In addition, lack of exercise is an independent risk factor for poor cholesterol, diabetes, high blood pressure, and being overweight, which are all additional risk factors for heart disease. Therefore, exercise can give you significant health benefits in multiple ways.

ALERT

The risk of being active is much smaller than the risk of being inactive. For that reason, the American College of Sports Medicine recommends that even people who are frail and/or elderly participate in some sort of regular physical activity. Do not let the tiny risk of an exercise-related injury outweigh the tremendous benefit.

The really great news is that research confirms that regular moderate-intensity exercise—at a minimum of thirty minutes a day on most days of the week—can have a powerful impact on improving your health. Moderate-intensity exercise includes activities like a brisk walk, fast enough that you break into a sweat but can still talk easily. To accumulate your thirty minutes of activity, you don't even have to do it all at once. People still enjoy improvements in health from as little as ten minutes of activity in three cumulative bouts over the course of the day.

High LDL Cholesterol

A high LDL (or bad cholesterol) level increases your risk of heart disease. Everyone should have an LDL of lower than 160mg/dl, but if you have several risk factors, your LDL should be far lower than that.

The risk factors that help determine your LDL goals are:

- Smoking
- High blood pressure (140/90mmHg) or on blood pressure medication

- Low HDL
- Family history of early heart disease (in the fifties or younger)
- Men forty-five and older or women fifty-five and older (postmenopausal)

According to the most recent government guidelines, ideal LDL cholesterol levels depend on how many other risk factors that you have. For example, if you have one or no other risk factors, your LDL cholesterol level is considered high if it is greater than 160mg/dL. It is considered "borderline high" if it is greater than 130mg/dL.

If you have two or more risk factors, your LDL cholesterol level is considered high if it is equal to or greater than 130mg/dL. If you have coronary artery disease or other equivalents (such as diabetes, peripheral arterial disease, symptomatic carotid artery disease, or an abdominal aortic aneurysm), your LDL cholesterol level is considered high if it is greater than 100mg/dL.

If your LDL cholesterol is in the borderline-high or high category, try to make some changes in your diet and increase your activity levels to lower your cholesterol. If you lower your cholesterol levels, you will reduce your risk of heart disease. Most coronary heart disease is caused by atherosclerosis, which occurs when cholesterol, fat, and other substances build up in the walls of the arteries that supply blood to the heart. Since atherosclerosis is a slow-progressing disease, you may not experience any symptoms for many years, possibly until it is too late. Lowering your LDL level will slow plaque buildup in the arteries and reduce your risk of disability or of a future heart attack or stroke.

Low HDL Cholesterol

Low levels of HDL, or good cholesterol, are considered a risk factor, since HDL cholesterol helps to prevent the buildup of cholesterol in the arteries. If you recall the liver manufacturing plant from Chapter 1, you will remember that HDL cholesterol gathers up free-floating cholesterol in the arteries and returns it to the liver. Low HDL levels mean there are fewer transports available to clean up the arteries. An HDL cholesterol level of less than 40mg/dL is considered low. An HDL of more than 60mg/dL is optimal.

Two steps you can take to raise levels of HDL cholesterol are to increase physical activity levels to a minimum of thirty minutes on most days of the week and, if you smoke, to quit.

Unmanaged Stress

Strong research evidence exists to support the negative effects of prolonged stress on health. While the government does not include unmanaged stress as a specific risk factor in the new cholesterol-management guidelines, numerous studies have demonstrated that chronic feelings of anger and hostility increase the risk of heart disease and hypertension.

Physical symptoms of stress include increased blood pressure and heart rate, chronic muscle tension, indigestion, irritability, anxiety, and altered sleeping habits, among other things. Reducing stress can minimize or eliminate these symptoms, which can improve your overall feelings of well-being. Furthermore, unless you manage the stress in your life, it is very difficult to successfully change any of your lifestyle habits.

The good news is that some health-enhancing activities, such as adding regular physical activity into your routine, also help to manage stress, improve heart health, and increase levels of good cholesterol.

Putting the Pieces Together

If you have high blood pressure and you also have high cholesterol levels, your risk of having heart disease increases six times. If you have high blood pressure, high cholesterol levels, and you are also a smoker, your risk of having heart disease increases by a factor of twenty. In other words, when you combine risk factors, the chance of developing cardiovascular disease is far more severe.

Notice that many of the risk factors can be reduced through the same methods:

- Physical Exercise
- Healthier Eating
- Quitting Smoking
- Reducing Stress

Not only do these methods reduce various risk factors, they also improve your cholesterol profile. In other words, by following these basic practices, you'll get the best results for your effort. These activities will be discussed in detail in future chapters.

CHAPTER 4

Know Your Numbers: Cholesterol Testing

The reason for testing your cholesterol levels is to understand your risk for developing heart disease, stroke, or any of the other consequences of atherosclerosis. Poor cholesterol has no visible symptoms. The only way to learn whether your cholesterol levels place you at risk for a heart attack or stroke is to measure your levels. You can get your cholesterol levels tested in your medical doctor's office, at a medical laboratory, or at public screenings.

When to Check Your Cholesterol Levels

Although cholesterol levels alone are not predictive of heart disease in all people, knowing your levels is a valuable first step toward understanding your risk status. When you know your cholesterol levels, as well as the status of your other risk factors, you gain valuable insight into the health of your current lifestyle and what you need to do to become or stay healthy. Furthermore, for those people who learn that they fall into high-risk categories, the sooner they begin a treatment plan to lower levels of bad cholesterol and increase levels of good cholesterol, the sooner they can start to reduce their risks of heart attack or stroke.

Cholesterol Testing for Healthy Adults

Federal government guidelines recommend that all Americans check their cholesterol levels with a complete fasting lipoprotein profile at the age of twenty. The measurements taken by this test include your levels of total cholesterol, HDL cholesterol, LDL cholesterol, and triglycerides. If test results indicate that all levels are in a healthy range, then government guidelines recommend retesting at a minimum of every five years. The full lipoprotein profile test is preferred over a test that provides data regarding only total cholesterol and HDL levels because knowing LDL cholesterol and triglycerides allows medical providers to better target adjustments in lifestyle and medical therapy. Regular blood pressure screenings, blood sugar checks, and physical exams are also recommended to better screen your overall health and cardiovascular risk.

FACT

If you do not fast at least nine to twelve hours before testing your cholesterol, you can measure only total cholesterol and HDL levels. To receive more detailed information regarding your levels of LDL cholesterol and your triglycerides, fasting is necessary. The reason for fasting is that certain foods and alcohol will cause your cholesterol levels to spike, making your cholesterol levels more dependent on the time and content of your recent ingestion rather than your body's composition.

Although federal government guidelines recommend cholesterol testing for adults at least every five years, if you have had a major change of lifestyle during that five-year period, your cholesterol levels may be different and, therefore, worth checking again before five full years elapse. For example, if you were a college student at age twenty and then became a working professional after graduation at age twenty-one or twenty-two, your physical activity levels, dietary choices, and stress levels may have changed significantly. All of these factors can impact your cholesterol levels. Therefore, it may be worth your time and effort to know your numbers as a measure of your health status in your new lifestyle. In general, you should err on the side of caution and get your levels checked more often. Cholesterol testing is relatively quick and inexpensive and reveals very valuable information.

Under current government guidelines, if you fall into a category that requires treatment for your cholesterol levels, you will have your cholesterol tested at much more frequent intervals to evaluate the success of the treatment program and to make any necessary adjustments. For example, if your health care provider suggests that you adopt therapeutic lifestyle changes, the follow-up visit and test should be within six weeks. If your health care provider suggests drug therapy, the initial follow-up visit and test should also be within six weeks. Subsequent visits for additional monitoring and adjustment of therapy should be scheduled at appropriate intervals depending on the nature of the individual therapy. Typically, if your cholesterol is in the borderline dangerous range, you should have a recheck in approximately six months. How often you receive subsequent rechecks will be based on your levels during the initial recheck and the opinion of your medical provider.

Cholesterol Testing for Children

Evidence from research shows that atherosclerosis often starts in childhood and can lead to cardiovascular disease in those as young as their twenties to forties. In families that are high-risk, it's even more important that from two years of age onward that children follow a healthy lifestyle that includes a nutritious low-fat diet and regular physical activity.

Cholesterol testing could also be the right motivation for a child of healthy weight to improve eating and exercise habits. Many kids who are not overweight do not make healthy choices and feel that they can get away with eating whatever they want. Since thin people also have heart disease, a concrete result of high cholesterol could motivate a thin child and family to make healthier eating and exercise choices. This would prevent both future disease and the risk of eventually becoming overweight.

ALERT

All children can benefit from adopting healthy habits in their youth. These habits include eating a diet low in saturated fats, cholesterol, and trans fats; participating in regular physical activities; and keeping weight at healthy levels. The greatest benefit is seen in children from families with a high risk of heart disease.

Since only half of adults who are overweight were overweight as children, this means that a lot of these thinner kids will become overweight in adulthood if they don't change their unhealthy eating and exercise habits. Families that make changes now will reduce cardiovascular complications in the long run.

Circumstances That Can Affect Your Test Results

Your general health also has an effect on your cholesterol test results. Do not go ahead with a scheduled cholesterol test if you have a cold or the flu. Cholesterol levels can go up or down temporarily during periods of acute illness, immediately following a heart attack or stroke, or during acute stressors such as surgery or an accident. For a more accurate measure, medical experts recommend that you wait at least six weeks after any illness before checking your cholesterol levels.

Your cholesterol levels reflect your lifestyle and your genetics. The ideal time to obtain an accurate test is when you are observing your usual routine. Cholesterol levels may change daily in response to deviations from your normal physical activity and eating habits, particularly if you increase your fat intake. Rapid weight loss also impacts cholesterol levels. These fluctuations in cholesterol do not occur immediately, but there is a definite response. Experts estimate that cholesterol levels may change by as much as 10 percent from one month to another simply from normal variations in metabolism. Therefore, for the truest insight into your risk of heart disease on the basis of your cholesterol levels, schedule your test at a time when you are living your typical, routine lifestyle.

Cholesterol Testing in Women

During pregnancy, women's cholesterol levels typically escalate. Unless your health care provider advises you differently, an increase from your typical cholesterol levels at this time is not usually a cause for concern. Medical experts recommend that women wait at least until six weeks after delivery before checking cholesterol levels.

In some women, removal of the ovaries may trigger an increase in cholesterol levels due to the subsequent hormonal changes. Menopausal women usually experience an increase in cholesterol levels, also likely related to reduced levels of estrogen. Be sure to discuss any changes in your typical cholesterol levels with your health care provider. See Chapter 15 for more information about special considerations for women with high cholesterol.

Influence of Prescription Drugs

Certain prescription medications may also lead to an increase in cholesterol levels. These medications include the following:

- ACTH (adrenocorticotrophic hormone)
- Anabolic steroids
- Beta-adrenergic blocking agents (beta blockers)
- Corticosteroids
- Epinephrine
- Oral contraceptives
- Phenytoin
- Sulfonamides
- Thiazide diuretics
- Vitamin D

If you are taking any medications that have a potential adverse impact on your cholesterol levels, be sure to discuss this with your health care provider. Make sure that you understand how you will monitor your cholesterol levels over time to ensure they remain within a healthy range.

Your Blood Cholesterol Test

When you have your cholesterol tested, you should have the full lipid profile. The results of this test include your levels of HDL (or good cholesterol), LDL (or bad cholesterol), and triglycerides. For accurate results, you need to fast for nine to twelve hours before the test. That means you may have nothing to eat or drink but plain water during that time. It is important that you do not consume any alcoholic beverages, coffee, tea, or soda—only drink water.

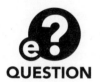

QUESTION

Why is it so important for me to fast before a lipid profile test?
The reason it is important not to eat for several hours before testing is that after a meal, triglycerides spike. To account for this variability and establish standards, studies of risk and therapy have been based on fasting cholesterol levels, as this gives the most reliable description of the body's current blood cholesterol composition.

What to Expect

Since you need to obtain a fasting profile, schedule your test for first thing in the morning. Your health care professional will take a blood sample, either from a vein or from a finger stick. After the health care provider has collected the blood, he or she will either send it to a lab for analysis or—if the test is being performed via a finger stick—a portable testing device will be used to analyze the sample.

If you are on any medications that affect cholesterol levels, such as those listed in Chapter 13, work with your health care provider to determine whether you should not take your prescription for a certain period of time before you take your cholesterol test.

Other Ways to Check Your Cholesterol

You may find public screenings for cholesterol at health fairs, your place of business, or at community events. These are becoming increasingly common as portable cholesterol screening has become easier, with results often given in minutes. Typically, technicians at screenings use a finger-stick sample and a portable testing device to measure test results. This test can provide you with accurate and valuable information.

Why Are Public Screenings Held?

Many different groups offer public screenings. Sometimes companies will offer cholesterol screenings for their employees in an effort to maintain the health and wellness of their staff. Public health organizations will often hold events as well to increase cholesterol awareness and educate the public on the importance of knowing one's cholesterol levels. Sometimes pharmaceutical companies will offer cholesterol screening in an effort to find people whose cholesterol levels may be in a higher-risk range and therefore may warrant pharmaceutical therapy. Typically, there is no harm to taking advantage of such screenings, as they do not commit you to any future obligation.

Blood Donation

Free blood cholesterol testing during blood donation is becoming increasingly common. Often blood donor centers are affiliated with hospitals that have laboratories that can easily perform such testing. The testing is typically offered as a thank you to blood donors and to increase overall cholesterol screening. Cholesterol testing is always optional and results will never disqualify blood donors from donating. Like public screenings, blood donation screenings may include only total cholesterol rather than a full lipid profile.

The Value of Public Screenings

The information you get from public screenings may be of limited use. First, since screenings typically occur in informal settings and without advance notice, you will have not fasted the recommended twelve hours prior. Also, certain testing machines are slightly less accurate than others, and public screenings may use more inexpensive, less accurate technology. Lastly, you may not receive a full cholesterol profile and therefore not know the full picture of your cholesterol health.

Your health care provider can provide help with interpreting any results, so share your test results with him or her if you have your cholesterol tested at a public screening. Even if you are able to take only a nonfasting total cholesterol and/or HDL test, it may provide you with helpful information. Keep a record of your results. If it is available, make sure that you obtain the fasting, full lipoprotein profile.

The greatest value of public screenings for cholesterol is in raising awareness of the prevalence of heart disease among the public. Public screenings help people realize that they are in need of further testing and evaluation. One of the greatest risks to your health is a lack of knowledge. Remember, the best method to deal with serious illnesses like a heart attack or stroke is prevention. Also, remember that cholesterol, like blood pressure and diabetes, can be a silent killer, as you have no way of feeling if your cholesterol levels are harmful.

Can You Know Too Much?

Cholesterol, like many basic measures of health, can vary on a day-to-day basis. It is possible to check too frequently and react too hastily to results. Remember, an appropriate screening has you fasting for at least nine to twelve hours, and even when done appropriately, there remains some variability. When one becomes overconsumed with measuring parameters of health, whether cholesterol, blood pressure, or blood sugar, one adds to the body's stress levels, which may worsen all of these measures. As you know, stress is a risk factor not only for a poor cholesterol profile but also is an independent risk factor for high blood pressure, high blood sugar, and cardiovascular disease itself. Therefore, you do not want to act in any way that is going to add stress to your life.

While testing and being informed are important, far more important are your actions to improve your health, no matter what your test results are. These tests offer only some idea of the relative impact these essential actions will have. If one focuses too much on the tests and loses sight of the goals of improving health and avoiding serious disease, then the testing becomes meaningless. Like any aspect of your health, the most important thing is finding the right balance.

CHAPTER 5

What Your Test Results Mean

Once you get your cholesterol screened, you receive a report with various figures, a ratio, and possibly a risk interpretation. It's not enough simply to know your numbers—you need to know what those numbers mean, and if you should take action to change your numbers. This chapter gives you insight into how to interpret your results in each of the following categories: total cholesterol, LDL cholesterol, HDL cholesterol, triglycerides, and ratio of total cholesterol to HDL cholesterol.

Total Cholesterol Results

In general, the higher your total blood cholesterol level, the greater your risk of heart disease. For example, a person with a total cholesterol level of 240mg/dL may have as much as twice the risk of heart disease as someone with a total cholesterol level of less than 200mg/dL.

Total cholesterol alone, however, does not tell the complete story. Heart disease risk is related to the composition of your total cholesterol. For example, if you have high total cholesterol due to a very high HDL cholesterol level, then that is a positive condition. On the other hand, if your total cholesterol is not high, but you have a high LDL level or a low HDL level, then that is a negative condition. Unfortunately, for most people, having a high total cholesterol means they have a high LDL level. Rarely will high total cholesterol be due to high HDL. This is why high total cholesterol likely means you are at higher risk for heart disease. Keep in mind, though, that as many as 50 percent of people who have heart disease do not have elevated lipid levels. For a more complete picture of your potential risk, you need to check your other lipid levels and consider your lifestyle habits and genetic history.

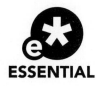

ESSENTIAL

Research shows that high levels of total cholesterol are indicators of future heart problems. Total cholesterol, however, is composed mostly of LDL particles. Therefore, leading experts believe that the strong relationship between total cholesterol and heart disease is reflective of the fact that high LDL levels are a risk factor.

Those who have cholesterol levels between 200 to 239mg/dL are considered to have borderline-high risk. However, this is not necessarily cause for alarm. If total cholesterol levels are high because of high HDL levels of more than 60mg/dL, it actually means that you have a reduced risk of heart disease, assuming that you have no other risk factors.

People with total cholesterol levels of 240mg/dL and above are classified as "high risk." Levels this elevated are almost always due to LDL. People in this category are at high risk of having a heart attack or stroke. They should implement aggressive lifestyle changes and possibly begin pharmaceutical treatments. Often those in this category warrant other cardiovascular testing as well.

Children and Adolescents

Scientific studies show that atherosclerosis, the building of obstructive plaques within arteries, actually begins in childhood. The federal government and the American Heart Association recommend the following guidelines on blood cholesterol in children and adolescents from the age of two to nineteen years:

▼ **CLASSIFICATION OF TOTAL CHOLESTEROL LEVELS FOR CHILDREN AND ADOLESCENTS**

Total Cholesterol Level	Category
Less than 170mg/dL	Acceptable
170–199mg/dL	Borderline
200mg/dL and above	High

Medical experts recommend cholesterol testing for children from families with a history of early heart disease or known cholesterol genetic disorders. Remember, cholesterol is a silent killer and the best method is prevention. For those with a particularly high risk, the earlier screening and intervention takes place, the more likely a heart attack or stroke can be prevented.

The majority of deaths from heart disease occur in older adults, simply because the disease has had more time to develop. Plaque has time to grow larger in blood vessels and cause more obstruction to blood flow. The challenge for older adults is that risk assessment by standard risk factors is less reliable, particularly as it is expressed as a percentage of risk over a ten-year period. This, however, does not mean that high total cholesterol levels in older adults should go untreated. Instead, remember that elevated cholesterol levels in older adults simply do not have the same predictive power as they do for other adults. As discussed, most large cholesterol-risk studies have been done on groups of middle-aged white males. However, more research is showing that the risk posed by elevated levels of LDL cholesterol and triglycerides does not discriminate based on age, gender, race, or any other demographic.

LDL Cholesterol Results

High levels of LDL cholesterol are known to be a major cause of heart disease. Federal government guidelines focus on reducing LDL levels as the primary means of providing therapy for people with high cholesterol. Strong research evidence supports the idea that reducing LDL levels results in reducing the risk of heart disease. However, before you assume that you have very high levels of LDL cholesterol based on the results of one test, make sure that you fasted for the recommended minimum of nine hours before you took your cholesterol test. If your LDL result was high and you are not certain you observed the fasting requirement closely, it's a good idea to repeat the test.

LDL Guidelines for Adults

The following table reflects the classification of LDL cholesterol levels that are recommended by both the federal government and the American Heart Association for adults.

▼ CLASSIFICATION OF LDL CHOLESTEROL LEVELS FOR ADULTS

LDL Cholesterol	Category
Less than 100mg/dL	Optimal
100–129mg/dL	Near optimal
130–159mg/dL	Borderline
160–189mg/dL	High
Above 189mg/dL	Very high

Current treatment approaches for people with high total cholesterol levels are based on LDL levels, other risk factors, and the calculated percentage of short-term risk of having heart disease. People with elevated cholesterol levels are classified into three categories of risk for treatment.

An existing diagnosis of coronary artery disease or an equivalent condition is a very important factor that affects the treatment goal for LDL-lowering therapy. If the following conditions are present, the individual is considered to fall into the highest category of risk and is therefore recommended to receive the most aggressive therapeutic treatment to achieve an LDL of less than 100mg/dL or lower:

- Known coronary artery disease
- Other forms of cardiovascular disease, such as peripheral arterial disease, abdominal aortic aneurysm, and symptomatic carotid artery disease
- Diabetes
- Two or more other risk factors

These other risk factors include:

- Smoking
- Age: males over forty-five years old or females over fifty-five years old
- Having a first-degree relative with premature heart disease (males over fifty-five years old, females over sixty-five years old)
- Hypertension

If you have only one of the Framingham risk factors without coronary artery disease or one of its equivalents, you are in the moderate-risk category and your recommended LDL is less than 130mg/dL. If you have none, then you are considered low-risk and want to maintain an LDL level below 160mg/dL, the cutoff for high cholesterol.

To summarize, if you are without any risk factors, you are considered low-risk and your LDL goal is 160mg/dL. If you have one of the risk factors of age, smoking, low HDL, high blood pressure, or a family history of premature heart disease, you are at moderate risk and your LDL goal is 130mg/dL. If you have two of these risk factors or if you have diabetes, coronary artery disease, or its equivalent, you are high-risk and your LDL goal is 100mg/dL or lower.

These recommendations are not absolute. New, slightly adjusted recommendations are constantly being proposed and fine-tuned. Your health care provider may further subclassify you and your risk and individually tailor your treatment goals and therapy. These guidelines are meant to give you a general idea of your cardiovascular risk and cholesterol goals.

LDL Guidelines for Children and Adolescents

Levels of LDL have a genetic correlation. Certain genetic disorders predispose young people to extremely high levels of LDL, which leads to a high risk of cardiovascular disease.

The recommended levels of LDL cholesterol in children differ slightly from the guidelines for adults. The following chart sets forth how various levels of LDL cholesterol are categorized in children:

▼ **CLASSIFICATIONS OF LDL CHOLESTEROL LEVELS IN CHILDREN AND ADOLESCENTS**

LDL Cholesterol Levels	Category
Less than 110mg/dL	Acceptable
110–129mg/dL	Borderline
Above 129mg/dL	High

For children, the government guidelines recommend lifestyle changes as the main therapeutic intervention, with decisions about medications often deferred until adulthood. These changes include improving eating habits and increasing physical activity. Since children typically lack other risk factors, if successfully implemented these changes will usually lead to desired LDL levels.

Older Adults and LDL Cholesterol

Clinical studies show that older adults respond effectively to therapies targeting LDL cholesterol levels. The same recommendations for reducing LDL cholesterol levels that apply to young and middle-aged adults also apply to older adults. Recommended therapies include both changes in lifestyle habits and use of prescription drugs if indicated.

HDL Cholesterol Results

Levels of HDL, or good cholesterol, show an inverse relationship to heart disease risk. Remember, HDL cholesterol acts as the transporter that takes cholesterol away from the blood vessels and back to the liver for metabolizing. Unlike LDL cholesterol and triglycerides, where high numbers mean increased risk, higher levels of HDL cholesterol mean a lower risk of heart disease. There are more transporters taking cholesterol away from the arteries, leading to less plaque buildup and clogging. In healthy individuals, HDL cholesterol represents approximately 20 to 30 percent of total cholesterol levels. Since HDL is only a minor fraction and has a narrower range, elevated total cholesterol typically is due to elevated LDL cholesterol and is considered a risk factor for cardiovascular disease.

FACT

Researchers have found that some individuals whose lower levels of HDL are due to genetic disorders also have a higher risk of heart disease. Again, genes can influence risk of heart disease, and they show why family history is important in determining your own risk.

Some scientists believe there are possibly multiple subtypes of HDL cholesterol, just as there are multiple subtypes of LDL cholesterol, and that some subtypes of HDL have more beneficial characteristics than others. As with LDL, in the future you may see more HDL subtype testing. For now, you know that in general elevated HDL is a negative risk factor, or something that lowers one's chance of developing cardiovascular disease.

HDL Cholesterol in Adults

A risk to health arises when HDL levels are too low. Evidence from studies shows that low HDL cholesterol is an independent risk factor for heart disease. This means that regardless of whether other risk factors are present, the risk of heart disease is higher for people with low HDL cholesterol. This is why HDL is a listed risk factor in determining the need for LDL therapy. A 1 percent decrease in HDL levels is associated with a 2 to 3 percent increase in heart disease risk. The following chart sets forth the classification of HDL cholesterol levels as adopted by federal government guidelines and the American Heart Association:

▼ **CLASSIFICATION OF HDL CHOLESTEROL LEVELS FOR ADULTS**

HDL Cholesterol Levels	Classification	Risk Category
Less than 40mg/dL	Low HDL cholesterol	High risk
40 to 59mg/dL	Moderate HDL cholesterol	Higher levels are desirable
60mg/dL and above	High LDL cholesterol	Negative risk factor

Interestingly, adult women tend to have higher HDL cholesterol levels than adult men, likely due to hormonal influences. According to government estimates, approximately one-third of all adult men and one-fifth of adult women have low HDL cholesterol levels that put them at increased risk of heart disease. At 40mg/dL, however, both men and women are considered to have low HDL—there is no separate recommendation for women. Nor is there a separate recommendation regarding HDL levels for children.

Natural strategies to increase HDL cholesterol include losing weight, increasing activity, and quitting smoking. Of these, exercise seems to have the most significant effect on HDL. These natural strategies have positive effects, including boosting energy and increasing strength, as opposed to the harmful side effects created by some prescription drugs.

ESSENTIAL

Some medications that lower LDL cholesterol also raise HDL levels, giving twice the bang for the buck. Medications, of course, come with their own risks, so be sure to discuss these risks with your doctor.

The Lipid Triad

Low amounts of dense HDL cholesterol tend to occur in association with the presence of small, dense LDL cholesterol and high levels of triglycerides. The relationship among these three types of lipids is known as the "lipid triad." Low HDL levels also tend to occur in conjunction with metabolic problems associated with insulin resistance. Many people who have the lipid triad also have Type 2 diabetes, creating the "metabolic syndrome."

Several factors can lead to low HDL cholesterol levels. Many are variables related to lifestyle factors and can be changed by adopting healthy habits. These factors include high triglycerides, excess weight, lack of physical activity, cigarette smoking, very high carbohydrate-intake levels (more than 60 percent of total calories per day), heredity, and drugs such as beta-blockers, anabolic steroids, or progestational agents.

Approximately 50 percent of people who have low HDL levels have a genetic basis for their condition. Some of these people have a type of low HDL cholesterol known as "isolated low HDL," so called because it does not appear as part of the lipid triad. All people, however, can change their HDL levels by improving their lifestyle habits, whether there is a genetic basis for the HDL or not. It's easy to see why making an effort to eat more healthfully, not smoke, and engage in activity on a regular basis is truly worth your time and energy. In addition to helping you improve your cholesterol, you will also lose weight and improve your blood pressure, greatly decreasing the chance of dying or becoming limited or paralyzed from a heart attack or stroke.

High HDL—A Negative Risk Factor

Research shows evidence connecting high HDL cholesterol levels with a lower risk level for heart disease. For this reason, high HDL levels are considered a negative risk factor. The use of this terminology can be confusing. Risk factors are known to be those conditions that increase the level of risk for heart disease. So what does it mean for a risk factor to be negative?

What this term refers to is the fact that high HDL cholesterol is such a positive condition that it actually "negates" one of the other risk factors. If you think of a regular risk factor as adding points to your risk score, a negative risk factor is one that gives you negative points, or subtracts points from your score. For example, having elevated HDL cholesterol might cancel out the risk from having elevated blood pressure. For this reason, high HDL levels are very important for maintaining a healthy heart and circulatory system. Despite "canceling" the risk, individuals can reduce their risk the most by having elevated HDL with no other risk factors. Remember, even with no risk factors there is still a significant chance of developing a heart attack or stroke, as these are the number one and two killers, respectively. Having risk factors makes you higher-risk, but having no risk factors does not take away risk. You just become lower-risk. Ideally, you should strive to eliminate harmful risk factors and maintain levels of elevated HDL cholesterol.

Triglyceride Results

Triglycerides are a form of fat. Their structure is made up of three fatty acids attached to glycerol. Triglycerides are present in most fatty foods and are the most common fat in the body. Triglycerides that float in the bloodstream provide fuel for energy when your sugar stores run low. Those that are not used for fuel are stored in the body's fatty tissues. Recent research has made it clear that high triglyceride levels are a marker for increased risk of heart disease and are possibly an independent risk factor. In addition, high triglycerides are usually present when other risk factors, such as diabetes and high LDL cholesterol, are present. Triglycerides make up a main component of VLDL, or very low-density lipoprotein. Like LDL, these low-density lipoproteins can form atherosclerosis and plaques and cause the same health risks.

Classifications of Triglyceride Levels in Adults

As the role of triglycerides in the process of developing heart disease becomes clearer, experts support efforts to keep triglyceride levels low. The federal government and the American Heart Association have come up with the following guidelines regarding fasting blood levels of triglycerides in adults:

▼ **CLASSIFICATIONS OF TRIGLYCERIDE LEVELS**

Triglyceride Level	Classification
Less than 150mg/dL	Normal
150–199mg/dL	Borderline high
200–499mg/dL	High
Above 499mg/dL	Very high

As with low HDL and high LDL levels, behavioral factors are the root cause of high triglyceride levels. Excess weight and lack of physical activity are the most common causes. However, any of the following can be a factor: cigarette smoking; excess alcohol consumption; very high carbohydrate-intake levels (more than 60 percent of total calories per day); drugs such as beta-blockers, corticosteroids, estrogens, and protease inhibitors for HIV; heredity; or other diseases such as Type 2 diabetes, chronic renal failure, and nephrotic syndrome. Notice that many contributors on this list are the same contributors to poor HDL and LDL levels, as well as independent risk factors for cardiovascular disease itself. People who do not have any of these factors generally have triglyceride levels of less than 100mg/dL. As with LDL and HDL, the first course of action to lower triglyceride levels is to adopt lifestyle changes, including improved nutrition and increased physical activity.

Total Cholesterol and HDL Ratio

Since total cholesterol is primarily composed of HDL and LDL, for a quick estimation of risk, you can calculate your total cholesterol and HDL ratio. To do this, divide your total cholesterol number by your HDL number. This method is based on the fact that high HDL levels relative to your total cholesterol are generally predictive of a lower risk of heart disease. While this estimate can give you a rough idea of your cholesterol-level breakdown, it is not recommended as a test upon which to base therapeutic treatment.

Today, the American Heart Association uses absolute numbers for LDL and HDL cholesterol levels. They are more useful to physicians than the cholesterol ratio in determining appropriate treatment for patients. If you're interested in calculating your ratio, the classifications are as follows:

▼ CLASSIFICATIONS OF RATIO OF TOTAL CHOLESTEROL TO HDL

TC/HDL Ratio	Classification
3.5 to 1	Optimum
4.5 to 1	Desirable
5 to 1 and above	High

To apply the formula, let's take an example of a woman with a total cholesterol level of 200 and an HDL level of 50. Her ratio is calculated by dividing 200 by 50, to equal a ratio of 4 to 1. According to this rough measure, her cholesterol is in the desirable range, but for a more comprehensive understanding, it's necessary to look at the entire spectrum of blood lipid levels.

Keep in mind that all of these numbers are not your health. They are tools to give you a better picture of the composition of your blood, which ultimately affects the health of your arteries and your heart. No matter what the test or technology, you hold the power to improve your own health and to feel and be your best. Your choices make all the difference between a better and longer life, or a sick life and untimely death.

Other Tests

Typically, your health care provider will include a cholesterol test as part of a routine physical checkup. In addition to blood lipid tests, medical professionals may use other tests to achieve a full picture of the health of the heart and circulatory system. This is particularly important if you have other risk factors, since 50 percent of people with heart disease have "desirable" cholesterol levels.

Noninvasive Diagnostic Tests

Several of the tests doctors use to measure the function of the heart and the state of the arteries are noninvasive, meaning they are done without entering the body or puncturing the skin. Instead, medical professionals use different types of technology to look at the heart and arteries and to measure how well they are functioning. These tests are typically performed on those considered at higher risk for cardiovascular disease.

In the stress test, you exercise on a treadmill or a stationary bicycle to put your heart under stress. As you are exercising, medical professionals will administer tests to measure your heart's response to the stress and ensure your arteries are not so clogged that you do not have adequate blood flow to meet the demand. An electrocardiogram (EKG), which measures the electrical flow through your heart, monitors your heart during the test. The test involves putting electrodes on your chest that are connected to a machine, the electrocardiograph. The electrocardiograph prints out a record of how the heart is beating and reveals any irregularities. As you exercise, the printout shows whether your heart is able to meet the extra demand placed on it by the exercise.

Another method of stress testing uses a radioactive tracer that is injected intravenously. The tracer flows through the arteries. Medical professionals use special cameras to view the tracer's passage as it reveals the extent of openness or blockage of various blood vessels.

ALERT

Studies show that some diagnostic tests and procedures are not as accurate in women as in men. For example, an exercise stress test may show a false positive or negative, but this is more likely in a younger woman. Some doctors prefer other types of tests that are more diagnostically accurate for young women.

Due to certain physical conditions, some individuals cannot undergo the rigors of a stress test. In these cases, doctors use medications to stress the heart as if it were exercising. They then follow the flow of the tracer and assess the health of the heart and its coronary arteries.

An echocardiogram, also known as an "echo" test or EKG, uses sound waves to take a dynamic picture of the heart as it beats. An ultrasound transducer transmits high-frequency sound waves directed toward the heart.

The cardiologist analyzes this moving picture of the heart to evaluate its functioning. Echocardiography reveals the shape and thickness of the walls in the heart's chambers and the large veins and arteries of the heart, among other things.

Medical professionals also use echocardiography with stress tests, performing the echo before the stress test begins and immediately after it stops.

Magnetic resonance imaging (MRI) and computed tomography (CT) are other noninvasive tests. These tests uses a magnet and/or radiofrequency waves to read signals from the body's cells to create an image of the interior of the body. To take the test, the patient lies on a mobile examination table that moves through a large tube.

The cardiologist analyzes the MRI images and data to evaluate the blood supply to the heart muscle and to assess the function of the blood vessels. In certain CT scans, the image reader can see calcium from plaques within the arteries that feed the heart muscle blood and oxygen.

Invasive Testing

An angiogram is an invasive test used to measure the degree of blockage in blood vessels. It is considered the best way to detect narrowing of blood vessels, but due to the risk of the procedure, it is done only in very high-risk individuals. To perform an angiogram, the physician punctures a major artery and inserts a long plastic catheter up to a heart blood vessel. Then a dye is injected into the catheter to allow for observation of the heart blood vessels. The doctor observes the dye's progress on an X-ray machine to see how it flows through the vessels.

If the angiogram reveals a blockage, the doctor may perform an angioplasty, which involves clearing the blockage from the artery and then placing a hollow tube, called a stent, on the inside of the blood vessel to keep it open. If the blockage is so severe that the artery cannot be saved, surgery to create a bypass to the blocked vessel may be required.

Intravascular ultrasound (IVUS) uses sound waves to create a multidimensional image that shows the level of blood flow and plaque buildup inside the coronary artery. Medical professionals take images using a catheter with a transducer inside the artery itself. This can provide an extremely accurate view of the size of the vessel's opening and condition of the plaque and arterial walls, but this technology is still in the early stages of development.

FACT

Medical professionals can use intravascular ultrasound (IVUS) to plan or evaluate the success of an angioplasty and the placement of a stent. They can also use IVUS to plan or evaluate the success of a bypass surgery procedure.

Blood Tests

The presence of higher-than-normal levels of C-reactive protein (CRP) or highly specific CRP (hsCRP) in the bloodstream is nonspecific evidence of an infectious or inflammatory disease in the body. CRP is not indicative of the presence of a specific disease but simply that the body is fighting some form of infection or inflammation.

Strong evidence from research studies shows that CRP is also a marker for heart disease. Women with high CRP levels were five times more likely than women with low CRP levels to develop heart disease and seven times more likely to have a stroke or heart attack. Again, an elevated CRP does not give any specific information, nor does a normal CRP rule out disease. CRP may only raise or lower the chance that a disease is occurring.

The reason that CRP levels can be a marker for heart disease is related to the fact that damage to, or inflammation of, the interior lining of the arteries (referred to as the endothelial lining) precedes the formation of plaque. In other words, plaque collects in locations where there is damage to arterial walls. CRP can be evidence of this damage.

When LDL cholesterol combines with a substance known as apolipo-protein (a), the result is a compound known as Lp(a), which can increase a person's risk of heart attack or stroke.

Federal government guidelines describe Lp(a) as an emerging risk factor. Researchers believe that the presence of Lp(a) can increase the formation of blood clots and the formation of plaque by assisting LDL particles to attach to plaque buildups.

ESSENTIAL

Approximately 50 percent of people who have heart attacks do not have elevated cholesterol levels. These individuals, however, typically have higher levels of CRP, Lp(a), or other potential markers such as apo B, or homocysteine. As researchers continue to learn about the exact mechanisms of heart disease, more tests are developed to identify and measure these other risk factors and markers.

Genetics determines your levels of Lp(a) and even the size of the Lp(a) molecule itself. Lifestyle changes do not alter levels of Lp(a); instead, levels for most people tend to remain consistent over a lifetime, except for women, who will experience a slight rise in levels with menopause. Some physicians request testing of Lp(a) for patients who have a strong family history of premature heart disease.

Treatment for elevated Lp(a) includes niacin therapy and concentrating efforts on lowering LDL levels, because at lower levels, it is harder for LDL particles to attach to plaque buildup.

CHAPTER 6

Creating Your Healthy Lifestyle

According to the Centers for Disease Control and Prevention, about half of all deaths in the United States are linked to behaviors that are changeable. As people are living longer, this percentage is only increasing. In other words, most people can do simple things to prolong their lives. Perhaps even more important, you can add to your quality of life by avoiding heart attacks or strokes. By making healthy choices, you will live longer, enjoy a higher quality of life, feel better about yourself, have more energy, and reduce your risks of disease and disability.

The Power to Create Health

You've learned about cholesterol. You've learned about the risk factors. You've learned that you can take steps to improve your cholesterol levels and accordingly improve your overall health. All this knowledge is meaningless if not applied to improve your life or the lives of others. This chapter examines the importance of improving your health. This means understanding not only the individual pieces of the puzzle—like eating better or exercising more—but also how to fit them all together over a lifetime. The power of the whole, an integrated wellness lifestyle, is much greater than the sum of the parts.

ALERT

> In today's environment, if you don't have an aggressive strategy for eating whole foods and incorporating physical activities, it is easy to gain weight. Most easy-access foods are loaded with salt, fat, sugar, and other unhealthy substances. Similarly, it's much easier not to put any effort into exercise than to make the effort. In other words, if you go through modern life passively and do what is easiest and most convenient, your choices are likely to lead to premature death and disability.

The purpose of this chapter, therefore, is to give you insight into what it means to create a healthy standard of living. You may not realize how easy it is to be unhealthy. Similarly, you may find a healthy lifestyle easy once implemented. Regardless of how difficult the challenge of changing your life, the rewards of simple healthy living are worth the commitment and effort.

Change never happens overnight. You will examine a psychological model of the process of change and learn tips on how you can stay motivated. The following chapters will provide more specific practical information on what to eat, what to do, and how to implement other strategies that enhance your wellness.

What Science Can Teach Us

The great benefit of being alive today is that scientific research provides an almost complete picture of the mechanisms behind cholesterol, atherosclerosis, and heart disease. In the process of unraveling how the physical system develops disease, even more insight is gained into how to prevent, or at least to deter, the disease processes. People even one generation ago did not have the depth of knowledge and understanding now available about how actions affect health and longevity. Acting with the knowledge that those before have acquired honors those who made the effort to understand bodies, as well as those who did not have the opportunity to benefit from such knowledge.

What You Can Do

What science cannot change is that you are the bottom line. In other words, just as money cannot buy happiness, it cannot buy health. Yes, money can buy access to the best health care providers, to all the procedures and drugs that are available, and to minimally processed whole foods. But even the wealthiest person on the planet cannot simply buy his or her health. Health must be created through active effort.

The World Health Organization defines health as "a state of complete physical, social and mental well being, not merely the absence of disease or infirmity." This definition of health is very expansive. It supposes an optimal condition of being, rather than a minimal state of being disease-free. So instead of putting your focus on how to stop disease, consider for a moment the power of shifting your focus to how to create optimal health. You have the power to achieve it. All you need is the knowledge, which this book can help to provide, and the motivation, which comes from deep within yourself.

FACT

Health does not come in a bottle or pill. Your doctor cannot "make" you healthy. Only you can create your health on a daily, weekly, monthly, and yearly basis. Your health is a direct result of your way of living—eating, breathing, walking, sleeping, and embracing life.

The Hazards of Modern Living

One of the greatest ironies of modern living is that it is actually much easier to survive in a manner that contributes to poor health and chronic disease than it is to live a life of vibrant, vital health. The reasons for this are many and complex. Some of the factors of modern convenience are closely intertwined with the leading risk factors for heart disease.

Poor Eating Habits

The foods that are the easiest to obtain and the most plentiful are fast, high-fat, high-sugar, calorie-rich, highly refined processed foods. These foods are often nutrient-poor yet cheap and effortless to find. It takes more time and dedication to find and prepare natural, whole foods. Fortunately, more and more grocery stores and restaurants offering healthy fare are opening everywhere, but healthy living still takes effort. But the rewards of eating such health-enhancing foods are clear. You will live longer and feel better.

What you eat has a powerful influence over whether you create a healthy blood lipid profile that includes low LDL cholesterol, high HDL cholesterol, and low triglyceride levels. Research supports that eating a primarily plant-based diet that consists of a large proportion of minimally processed (or whole) grains, vegetables, and fruits is essential to support optimal health.

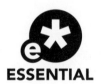

ESSENTIAL

The challenge of modern living is that it makes it very easy to overeat foods. Restaurant and fast-food portions are too big, and servings listed under nutritional information are too small.

Lack of Exercise and Excess Weight

Technology has made life so easy that it takes perseverance to find opportunities to move. Modern innovations have created so many labor-saving devices that the requirement to move is almost obsolete. This is not good for health. To create optimum health, the human body needs physical activity.

In the old days, people did not need to exercise because the tasks of daily living kept them active, whether walking several miles to do simple tasks or working in farm fields all day. In contrast, today you can drive to work or to run errands, sit in a chair to perform your job, shop and play games on your computer, use elevators and escalators to transport your body, and even use remote-control devices to operate the appliances in your home. Physical education is no longer a required daily curriculum for many children, and stationary, technology-driven activities are often children's choice for play instead of physical outdoor games.

All of this technology means that something people used to take for granted, such as walking around each day to complete tasks or even to have fun and play, is no longer an essential part of modern lives. Instead, people need to plan for movement. They need to brainstorm strategies to stay active. All of this inactivity has contributed to weight gain. When the inactivity is combined with easy-to-grab calorie-rich foods, even more weight gain is the result.

Exposure to Toxins

Another aspect of modern living that makes it difficult to support health is that you are exposed to environmental toxins, including numerous carcinogens. Cigarette smoke, air pollution, and other harmful chemicals in the air, water, and food supply undermine people's well-being. Scientific studies have also proved them harmful to both human health and to the environment.

ALERT

Chemicals and other toxins in the water, air, buildings, and food supply are impossible to avoid completely. Although you cannot totally control the environment you live in, you can do your part to minimize dangerous exposures, whether by not smoking, by filtering water, or eating whole foods.

Mental Stress

One of the most prominent features of modern living is the difficulty of escaping the mental stresses of daily life. Technology continues to drive the pace of work and living to faster and faster speeds. The cost of living, the pressure of competition for material wealth, and the challenge of balancing family, professional, and community ties all contribute to increasing daily pressures. Finding time to relax, unwind, and savor simple pleasures becomes a rare treat and often requires effort in itself.

In addition to the specific stress-related disorders that this daily pressure causes, stress makes it all the more challenging to actively pursue healthy eating and active habits. At the end of a long, hard day, it's much easier to grab a fast snack, sit on the couch, and do what you need to do to get through the rest of the day. It takes much more discipline and motivation to spend time meal-planning, shopping carefully, strategizing on how to be more active, and creating time to relax in refreshing and restorative ways.

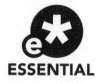

ESSENTIAL

Every step that you take toward positive living is good and valuable. Appreciate that it is challenging to create your healthy life, but know it is more than worthwhile to get pleasure from many years of feeling great, having energy, enjoying life, and being your best. Change may be hard, but it's not nearly as hard as death or a devastating illness.

One of the greatest dangers of stress is the damage it does to your body. Stress releases the chemical cortisol, which is known to raise LDL, lower HDL, and raise triglyceride levels, worsening your cholesterol profile in every way possible. Cortisol creates free radicals, which contribute to plaque formation. Stress also raises your blood pressure and blood sugar, creating even more risk for a stroke or a heart attack. Stress, like cigarette smoking, poor eating, and not exercising, increases your cardiovascular risk in multiple ways.

So what do you do? Start educating yourself about what a healthy lifestyle requires and the rewards and benefits of the extra effort that it is going to take. Start acknowledging that, all things being equal, it is more difficult to live a life that nurtures and supports your health in the short run, but living healthy will pay off tremendously in the long run. Be patient and gentle with yourself, and congratulate yourself for taking any time and making any effort in the direction you want to go. Remember that any effort you exert now will give you more energy and productivity and a longer life in the future. Also remember that while change is hard, once you change, continuing your healthy lifestyle will become easier.

The Process of Change

As you get ready to embark on your own path toward healthful living, it is useful to learn not only what to change, but how to change it. Behavioral-medicine researchers constantly examine how to support the process of change. Most people know they should eat more fruits and vegetables, exercise more regularly, decrease stress, and not smoke, so the question for scientists becomes, "Why aren't more people doing it?" Researchers realize that changing behaviors is a very difficult task, and they seek to understand how to improve the process to maximize people's odds of success.

A leading psychological model for behavioral change divides the course of action into five stages of readiness that are very useful for analysis. Understanding this progression can help you find success in achieving your goal of living a healthier lifestyle. The five stages include precontemplation, contemplation, preparation, action, and maintenance.

These phases are meant to describe the process of becoming more ready for change and, therefore, more likely to succeed. In other words, you must become truly ready and motivated to change a behavior first, before you start to take action. And, if the process is cultivated in that order—motivation first, action second—the odds of ultimate success in achieving lifestyle changes are much higher. Action without motivation may get things started, but it is simply not sustainable.

FACT

Not all people follow a linear path on the road to change. For example, a person may progress to the action stage and then return to the contemplation stage. What is important is that you continue to try—don't let your setbacks become permanent.

Precontemplation

Congratulations! Anyone who is reading this book has already progressed beyond the precontemplation stage. A person in the precontemplation stage is not making any behavioral changes and does not intend to make any changes. A person at this stage is not motivated and does not have the tools and information necessary to make a positive change.

This person feels it is easier to stay in his or her situation and even risk poor health and a shorter life than it is to make any changes. You may have friends or loved ones who are at this level. You, by reading this book, have chosen to take action and therefore have passed precontemplation.

Contemplation

In the contemplation stage, a person knows it is better to live a healthier lifestyle. Although the person is thinking about it, he or she has not yet taken any action toward making this change a reality. During this stage, a person is engaged in information-gathering and weighing the pros and cons of taking any action. This person has not yet made any commitment to change but is instead just thinking about it. This, however, is a very important stage.

If you feel you are in the contemplation stage, then you are doing exactly the right thing by reading and learning more about the benefits of making positive modifications toward a healthier lifestyle.

QUESTION

How can I help friends or loved ones who are in the contemplation stage?
The best way to provide support is to share information about specific benefits that come with adopting healthier behaviors. For example, tell them that a person who starts a moderate exercise program will sleep better at night and have more energy during the day. These are usually benefits everyone can relate to and wants to enjoy.

Preparation

People who are in the preparation stage have already started taking small steps toward acquiring new, healthy habits. For example, if a person plans more physical pursuits, she has gone out and bought a new pair of walking shoes. Or, if a person wants to eat more healthfully, he has purchased a book such as this one, full of heart-healthy recipes and tips for incorporating better snacking habits.

The best way to help someone who is in the preparation phase is to provide support and encouragement to continue to take action. Keep visual cues and props in obvious places. For example, post pictures of fruits, vegetables, whole grains, or fit and healthy role models on the refrigerator. Keep workout equipment, such as shoes, both at home and in the office as reminders. Persist in learning about all the benefits available from eating nutritious foods, staying active, managing stress, and feeling your best.

Action

In the action stage, things start to get exciting. This is the first six-month period of starting up a new exercise program, following a new eating pattern, or of integrating new methods of relaxation into your day. Studies show that it typically takes two months to develop a new habit and that as many as 50 percent of people who start a new program drop out within the first six months. Strategies to make it through the first six months include eliciting support from friends, family, and coworkers, and keeping useful reminders to continue doing your new routines and practices in places where you look frequently. The most important thing is using your motivation and contemplation to make sure you create the time and organize your life so you can sustain your newly developed habits.

Maintenance

The ideal conclusion to a concentrated effort in making a behavioral change is to reach the maintenance phase. In the example of incorporating regular activity, you get to the maintenance phase when you have exercised regularly for at least six months. By this point, you get used to the time and methods with which you exercise. Sustaining the behavior becomes much easier and self-motivating, because it is easy to feel the benefits and rewards of the healthy activity.

This does not mean it does not require effort to sustain the activity, so do not let your guard down. As always, being healthy will take effort and motivation. It's important to incorporate fun and different activities to keep motivation levels high, and the longer the behavior is continued, the less likely you are to drop it.

Dealing with Relapse

As the saying goes, humans are creatures of habit. Change is not easy. Relapsing is a normal part of the process. In fact, studies show that people who ultimately succeed in quitting smoking usually have tried to quit at least three times.

If you relapse, approach the process of change as a learning experience. With every step forward, figure out what worked. With every step backward, rather than beating yourself up, try to determine why that backward step occurred. If you approach transformation of your habits as a journey and as a self-learning adventure, you are likely to find more success. Remember to forgive yourself and keep on going.

ESSENTIAL

Your new health practices, such as eating a piece of fruit for breakfast or completing a set of push-ups in the morning, are not burdensome "problems" or "prescriptive medicines." View them as solutions that will improve your life, not another duty to add to your list of chores. Rather than thinking about the energy it's taking, think about the energy you are gaining.

Find ways to incorporate healthy habits that work for you so that you will continue to do them. For example, if you don't care for raisins, don't plan to eat them on your oatmeal every morning for breakfast. It will feel as if you are taking a nasty medicine that you hate. Instead, find something that you like to eat that is also good for you and plan to include more of it in your diet. Perhaps you enjoy blackberries or bananas or fruit salad or smoothies. Perhaps you enjoy swimming and basketball more than running or lifting weights. Maybe even a nicotine patch is enough to keep you from smoking—even that is a healthier alternative.

If you find that you need someone to help keep you accountable with your diet or in a regular exercise program, consult a registered dietitian or hire a personal trainer to work with on a regular basis. Enlist your friends and family. One of the best sources of motivation for anyone is not to want to let others down, even more than not wanting to let himself down. Set yourself up to win. Don't punish yourself. Reward yourself. Find solutions that work and make you feel good about you.

Believe in Yourself

Another important concept that researchers have determined is fundamental to successful change is how much you believe in your own ability to achieve it. Self-confidence is important. The more you believe you can achieve success, the more likely you are to find it. In contrast, if you see yourself as a person who simply can't eat nutritious foods or who can't possibly find time to move around more during the day, then it will come true for you. Your perception of yourself is powerful.

Furthermore, the power of your belief in yourself is behavior-specific. For example, you may have confidence you can walk at least thirty minutes most days of the week. At the same time, you may have far less certainty that you can eat more vegetables and less candy every day. You need to build your confidence in each particular area in which you want to succeed. Also, you need to believe that you can achieve the goals that you set for yourself.

Changing your thoughts, like anything else, requires active effort. It may mean paying more attention to your thoughts in general and, when you notice a negative one, escaping that thought pattern. You might distract yourself with other more positive thoughts or even pinch yourself to condition yourself away from self-defeating thinking. As with contemplation and motivation, you may find it possible to change your thoughts for the better by changing your environment with positive photos, exercise equipment, and the right foods.

Identify Your Priorities

Here's an interesting exercise to help you get in touch with what really matters in your life. Take a few moments to write down the top five things that are important to you. Examples of items you may want to include are your family, health, community, profession, a hobby, political causes, or volunteer work. Then, on the same piece of paper, list the top five activities that take up most of your time in an average day. Note the percentage of your waking time that they require.

Take a moment to compare how you spend your time each day with what you value most in your life. Have you found a good match? Or have you realized that you are neglecting some things that are very important to you? Once you increase your awareness of the way you are spending your time versus the way you want to spend your time, you can start making a difference. As you bring your unconscious habits and behavior patterns out into the open, you can begin realistically to assess small steps that you can take toward your new goals.

How can understanding your cholesterol help with spending more time on your priorities? With your cholesterol under control, and by following a sensible diet and exercise program, you'll have more energy, more time for activities, and a longer life to achieve your goals. You can take charge of your priorities by understanding and acting on your cholesterol.

For example, if you realize that you are spending three hours each day watching television and no time walking or participating in any other type of moderate physical activity, you can see that there is some time in your day that you can carve out to use for exercising. If you really can't give up your television time, then consider ways to do some exercises as you watch your favorite programs. Then, try to do this at least four days a week.

So consider how having more energy and a longer life span will allow you to give more time to some of those priorities, whether it be family, work, religion, or whatever else matters to you. Again, the investment in your health up front will pay handsome dividends in the future.

You May Have Just Saved a Life—Yours

Last, but certainly not least, remember to reward yourself for your good behavior. For example, promise yourself that if you stick to your new eating plan or exercise schedule for four consecutive weeks, or ideally six months, you will reward yourself with a nice massage or buy yourself some new exercise clothing. Of course the greatest reward will be how your new health will benefit you and your loved ones.

Living in a time when you can better understand your health and can strive to optimize your health is truly a privilege. When you move about, realize the joy of experiencing the sensation of your muscles in action. As you eat a dish of fresh foods, savor the flavors, colors, aromas and textures that whole foods add to your dining pleasure. And as you feel stronger, more energetic, and simply more alive, know that it is the direct result of your efforts to create a healthy life. You can do it—just keep believing in yourself and in your worth, because you are worth it.

CHAPTER 7

How to Eat!

What you put in your body directly creates your health. Your diet has been definitively associated with four of the ten leading causes of death in the United States—coronary heart disease, stroke, Type 2 diabetes, and certain cancers—and is likely linked to most of the other causes of death, as well. The foods you eat can increase or decrease your risk of heart disease, disability, and death. A diet that contributes to atherosclerosis is a major, modifiable risk factor, which means that you can make a powerful difference simply by choosing good foods.

You Are What You Eat

In its 2010 guidelines, the American Heart Association strongly endorses "consumption of a diet that contains a variety of foods from all the food categories and emphasizes fruits and vegetables; fat-free and low-fat dairy products; cereal and grain products; legumes and nuts; and fish, poultry, and lean meats." Researchers agree that food-based guidelines are more practical and easier to understand than those that focus on counting calories, fat, or cholesterol. These guidelines were initially issued over a decade ago and have continued to be reaffirmed by countless amounts of research.

FACT

The six major food groups are dairy; meats, eggs, and nuts; vegetables; fruits; grains; and fats, oils, and sweets. Within each food group, the goal is to select a variety of foods to ensure that you get all the essential nutrients you need.

The American Heart Association guidelines recommend the following foods:

- Five servings of fruits and vegetables a day
- Six servings of whole grains a day
- Two servings of fish per week
- May include lean meats and dairy

These guidelines are meant to emphasize the importance of choosing an overall balanced diet with foods from all major food groups, especially fruits, vegetables, and grains. In addition to including the recommended number of servings of the first three types of foods, include balanced amounts of the other foods listed in your meal choices.

The above guidelines are appropriate for everyone age two years and older. Laying the foundation for healthy eating patterns in children is critically important in helping them build healthy habits and in preventing the development of diseases later in life.

The Difference You Can Make

When scientists first began investigating the causes of heart disease, fats were identified as an enemy. However, as more and more research studies have determined, the picture is more complex than that. As with good and bad cholesterol, there are good fats and bad fats. The good fats are unsaturated fat, named for fats that are not "saturated" with high-energy hydrogen bonds. Specifically, the best, most heart-protective fats are called omega-3 and omega-6 fatty acids. They earned these names based on where a hydrogen bond is missing on the fatty-acid chain. These healthy fats are located more in produce, nuts, and fish oils. Researchers today support the concept that a primarily plant-based diet, including vegetable oils and fatty fish, is optimal for supporting health.

The Mediterranean Diet

Researchers became intrigued by the diet of southern Europeans (those who live near the Mediterranean) when they realized that people from this area enjoyed a very low incidence of heart disease and tended to live longer than North Americans and northern Europeans. The Mediterranean diet is characterized by a high intake of fruits and vegetables, nuts and cereals, and olive oil. In addition, fish is a regular feature. In contrast, the amount of meat and poultry consumed is minimal.

Though genetics may play a role, this better health does not seem to hold true for those from this area who immigrate to the United States and gorge themselves on a Western diet. In fact, controlled studies have shown that people placed on a Mediterranean diet can lower their chances of having another heart attack by almost two-thirds, no matter what their genetic background.

These studies confirm the power of dietary influences on heart health. What is even more interesting is that when the dietary components are examined, researchers have found that while following certain components benefits your health, following all components is much more powerful than the sum of their parts.

The Dietary Approaches to Stop Hypertension (DASH) Diet

The DASH diet similarly in emphasizes plant-based foods with lean meats and fish. DASH also focuses on lowering sodium intake. Investigators found that reductions in blood pressure with the DASH diet were as strong as any single medication. Again, the strongest effect was seen in those who ate plants and vegetables along with lean dairy and fish. They also reduced their LDL cholesterol levels 9 percent. In other words, the risk of heart disease could be reduced through dietary factors alone—not through supplements or any individual magic food, but rather through a dietary pattern that focused on a variety of whole, fresh foods that included calcium-rich foods.

Whether Mediterranean, DASH, or whatever "diet" you take on, the most important point is consistently eating fresh produce, whole grains, low-fat dairy, fish, and lean meats in moderation.

How Most of Us Eat

To achieve healthy cholesterol levels, the first course of action is to avoid foods that elevate LDL cholesterol. This priority comes from the evidence that high total cholesterol (from mostly high LDL cholesterol levels) increases the risk for heart disease and stroke. Lowering LDL cholesterol levels reduces these risks.

The Risk of Animal Foods

There is a direct relationship between the increased intake of saturated fatty acids, often called saturated fats, and an increase in LDL cholesterol levels. Saturated fatty acids are found in animal-based foods such as meats and dairy products. Steaks and chops, hamburger, sausage, processed meats (such as lunchmeat, hot dogs, or salami), and fatty cuts of meat are all common sources of saturated fats, as is the skin on poultry. Dairy products that are rich in saturated fat include cheese, butter, whole milk, 2 percent milk, ice cream, cream, and whole-milk yogurt. Plant-based foods typically do not contain any saturated fat.

For those who do not have heart disease or high levels of LDL cholesterol, the American Heart Association recommends that saturated fat intake represent less than 10 percent of total calories per day, and the less you consume, the better it is for your health. For those who have cardiovascular disease or high LDL cholesterol, the recommendation for daily consumption of saturated fat is much lower, less than 7 percent of total calories.

The following steps show an example of how a person without high cholesterol levels might determine his recommended daily amount of saturated fat. In this example, assume a daily recommended intake of calories, based on activity and metabolic needs, of roughly 2,000 calories per day.

1. Calculate the total number of calories from saturated fat, at less than 10 percent of total calories per day, as follows:

   10 percent (or .10) x 2,000 calories = 200

2. Next, calculate the total grams of saturated fat, at less than 10 percent of total calories per day, with the following formula:

   200 calories from saturated fat ÷ 9 calories per gram = 22.22

This person should consume less than 22g of total saturated fat per day.

The following steps show how to determine calories and grams for a diet with less than 7 percent saturated fats. This example would apply to a person with cardiovascular disease or high cholesterol levels and again assumes a diet of 2,000 calories per day.

1. Calculate the total number of calories from saturated fat, at less than 7 percent of total calories per day, as follows:
   7 percent (or .07) x 2,000 calories = 140
2. Next, calculate the total grams of saturated fat, at less than 7 percent of total calories per day, with the following formula:
   140 calories from saturated fat ÷ 9 calories per gram = 15.55

This person should consume less than 16g of total saturated fat per day. Again, the less saturated fat, the better. Although consuming moderate amounts of healthy fats may be good for your health, the negative impacts of consuming saturated fats far outweigh any positive impacts.

To see how those figures apply to a serving of real food, here's the breakdown for a cheeseburger. A three-ounce hamburger patty has approximately 7g of saturated fat. A 1-ounce piece of Cheddar cheese has 6g of saturated fat. One tablespoon of mayonnaise has approximately 2g of saturated fat. So far, this hamburger contains 15g of saturated fat, and we're not even finished putting it together! When you break down the numbers, it's easy to see how saturated fat grams add up quickly if you eat a lot of meat and dairy foods.

ALERT

The current consumption of saturated fats in the average American diet is 13 percent of total calories, in excess of the current recommendations for health. For some, it is much higher.

Since it is difficult or nearly impossible to analyze every bite of food that you put in your mouth, a good rule of thumb for limiting saturated fats in your diet is simply to reduce the amount of animal-based foods that you eat. See Chapter 8 for specific strategies to help reduce your intake of animal-based foods. When you choose more plant-based foods, you will naturally eat fewer animal-based foods. Plus, living without all those calculations is easier and makes mealtime a lot more pleasant.

Moving Away from Meats and Animal Fats

Trans-unsaturated fatty acids, often referred to as trans fats, are more harmful to your health than saturated fats and are the most harmful to your health in general of any type of fat. Trans fats earned the name based on the type of chemical bonds they have, called trans bonds. As with saturated fats, there is a direct relationship between an increased intake of trans fats and an increase in LDL cholesterol levels. Additionally, a direct relationship exists between increased consumption of trans fats and a reduction in HDL levels. Therefore, a diet high in trans fats does double damage, first by increasing your levels of bad cholesterol and second by simultaneously reducing your levels of good cholesterol. While saturated fat raises your LDL, it may raise or at least keep the same levels of HDL. Trans fats negatively affect all types of cholesterol.

Trans fats are artificially made and primarily found in commercially processed foods such as pies, doughnuts, cookies, chips, candy, pastries, shortening, and fried fast foods. Food manufacturers create trans fats through a process called hydrogenation that converts otherwise liquid oils into a more solid substance. This hydrogenation is useful to food manufacturers because it increases the shelf life of foods, adds form to otherwise liquid substances, and adds flavor. Studies, however, have confirmed that there is no level of consumption of trans fats that is considered safe. While minimizing your consumption of saturated fat is important, it is even more important to minimize, and ultimately eliminate, any consumption of trans fats.

Years ago, completely avoiding trans fat was difficult because it was found in so many foods. Now that its effect on cardiovascular disease continues to become more known, more manufacturers are eliminating trans fat from their products. Many products are advertised as "trans fat-free." This does not necessarily mean the product is healthy; it just means it is not as harmful. Paying close attention to other food contents remains worthwhile.

Research supporting the fact that there are no safe levels of trans fats in the diet is so strong that the U.S. Food and Drug Administration instituted a food-labeling requirement for trans fats in 2006. Food manufacturers are now required to list the amount of trans fats per serving in any food product.

There is a loophole in this labeling, though. Manufacturers can list 0g of trans fat as long as the content of trans fat is 0.49g or lower. Many feel this is a dangerous loophole, as serving sizes are often smaller than the portions you eat. This could potentially lead to further trans-fat consumption while you consume foods you believe are trans fat-free. This rounding to zero has even caught the attention of the World Health Organization, which has recommended people consume less than 2g of trans fat per day. Many people are possibly surpassing this mark without even knowing it, despite an effort to consume the ideal amount of 0g of trans fat. While legislators might pursue this in the near future, in the meantime, you should continue to consider how "natural" products are and look for terms such as "partially hydrogenated oils" on the ingredients list. If those sorts of artificial preservatives and flavorings are present, the food is more likely to contain at least some trans fat.

The good news is that food manufacturers are getting involved and responding to the evidence that these fats are so harmful to health. PepsiCo, one of the world's largest producers of commercial foods and beverages, has undertaken an initiative to eliminate trans fats from its snack products, which include popular lines such as Frito-Lay chips, Doritos, Lays, Ruffles, Cheetos, and Cracker Jack snacks, among others. When McDonald's eliminated trans fats from the oil used to make its French fries, that one small change was estimated to save tens of thousands of lives annually.

As food manufacturers and distributors become more aware that people care about food choices, they will make more healthful products available. Vote with your dollars and choose health and vitality. The length and quality of your life depends on it.

Cholesterol from Animal-Based Foods

Just as the cells in the human body contain cholesterol, so do the cells of all other animals. Plants and plant-based foods, however, contain no cholesterol. A good rule of thumb to remember is that many foods that are high in saturated fats are also high in cholesterol. Cholesterol-rich foods include organ meats (such as liver), certain shellfish, poultry, dairy products, and eggs.

Eating foods high in cholesterol can increase LDL cholesterol levels, but not nearly as much as eating foods high in saturated fats and trans fats can. In other words, you will improve your cholesterol levels more by cutting down on foods high in saturated and trans fats than by reducing consumption of foods that contain cholesterol. In general, though, foods high in saturated and trans fats are also high in cholesterol, so by reducing your consumption of those foods, you will reduce your consumption of several harmful substances. In other words, by moving away from animal-based foods, you get the most health for your effort.

The American Heart Association guidelines recommend an average daily consumption of dietary cholesterol of less than 300mg for healthy people. For people who know they have cardiovascular disease, diabetes, or elevated lipid levels, the recommendation is less than 200mg. Currently, the average daily consumption of dietary cholesterol in the United States is 256mg. The amount consumed among men is slightly higher, at 331mg, than it is for women, at 213mg. Therefore, the current average consumption of cholesterol-rich foods among the average healthy Americans is at appropriate levels to support health. Overconsumption, though, can lead to the many cardiovascular risks discussed previously.

▼ FOODS TO CHOOSE FOR A HEALTHY HEART

Foods to Choose More Often	Foods to Choose Less Often
Breads, Cereals, Rice, and Starches (6 servings or less per day, adjusted to caloric needs)	
Whole-grain breads, cereals, and pasta	Bakery products made with refined flour (doughnuts, croissants, sweet rolls, Danish)
Brown rice	Cakes, pies, coffee cakes, cookies
Potatoes	Biscuits, butter rolls, muffins
Dry beans and peas	—
Whole-grain crackers	Processed and refined grain–based snacks (chips, cheese puffs, snack mix, regular crackers, buttered popcorn)
Vegetables (3–5 servings per day)	
Fresh, frozen, or canned vegetables without added fat, sauce, or salt	Vegetables fried or prepared with butter, cheese, or cream sauce
Fruits (2–4 servings per day)	
Fresh, frozen, canned, or dried fruits, without added sugars	Canned fruits packed in heavy syrups
Dairy Products (2–3 servings per day)	
Fat-free, ½-percent or 1-percent milk, buttermilk, yogurt, cottage cheese	Whole milk, 2-percent milk, whole-milk yogurt
Fat-free and low-fat cheese	Regular ice cream, cream, cheese
Eggs* (no more than 2 egg yolks per week)	
Egg whites or egg substitute	Egg yolks, whole eggs
Meat, Poultry, Fish (5 ounces or less per day)	
Lean cuts of vegetarian-fed meats	Higher-fat meat cuts from animals fed animal-based foods
Loin, leg, round	Ribs, T-bone steak, bacon
Extra-lean hamburger	Regular hamburger
Cold cuts made with lean meat or soy protein	Cold cuts, salami, bologna, hot dogs, sausage
Skinless grain-fed poultry	Poultry with skin
—	Organ meats (liver, brains, sweetbreads)
Wild fish	Fried fish
Fats and Oils (amount adjusted to caloric needs)	
Unsaturated oils	Coconut oil
Soft or liquid margarines	Stick margarine
Vegetable oil spreads	Butter, shortening
Salad dressings, seeds, and nuts	—

*Recommendation for people with elevated lipid levels

How We Can Eat

Nutrition experts believe that the best way to achieve a healthy diet is to think in terms of what types of food to eat, rather than what to eliminate. It is much easier to focus on what you are eating than what you are not. They recommend that you keep in mind that the healthiest diet consists primarily of whole foods from plants, including grains, nuts, seeds, fruits, and vegetables. Focusing on a plant-based diet does not mean that you have to become a vegetarian. It simply means that the ideal diet to enhance health contains more plant-based than animal-based foods. Think about how humans evolved. For centuries, humans primarily survived off produce and grains in moderate amounts, because harvesting was always a challenge. People also ate fish, as evolving societies needed to be near water. Occasionally they would eat meat if there was a productive hunt, but this was a luxury, not a staple.

Fruits and Vegetables

Studies show that a high consumption of fruits and vegetables is associated with lower risks of developing heart disease, stroke, and hypertension. Unlike many high-fat and high-sugar processed foods, fresh fruits and vegetables are nutrient-dense and low in calories. Fruits and vegetables are also high in water content. This helps to maintain adequate hydration levels and helps you feel full. Eating these foods provides you with plenty of healthy fiber, essential nutrients, and beneficial phytochemicals and antioxidants.

Phytochemicals are chemicals that give plants colors and assist in keeping the plants healthy. In the same way that they fight disease, oxidation, and inflammation in plants, they can also further human health. Different phytochemicals support heart health through different protective actions. Antioxidants such as certain vitamins, carotenoids, and flavonoids prevent oxidation and decrease the likelihood of oxidized LDL cholesterol sticking to arterial walls. Recall that when LDL cholesterol is oxidized, it forms arterial plaque (as described in Chapter 1). Vitamins C and E are rich sources of antioxidants. Furthermore, it is preferred to obtain these antioxidants from foods, rather than from supplements.

Vegetables and fruits are also a rich source of the B vitamin complex.

Other minerals play a valuable role in regulating blood pressure and in keeping blood vessels healthy. Remember that another part of the atherosclerosis picture is that the walls of the blood vessels need to be inflamed or damaged before any arterial plaque can attach to them. Minerals such as calcium, magnesium, and potassium can help to keep these vessel walls healthy. As studies have shown, people who have healthier blood pressure levels tend to eat a diet full of fruits and vegetables that are rich in these nutrients. Food sources of calcium, magnesium, and potassium include artichokes, cantaloupes, broccoli, bananas, cauliflower, and bell peppers.

Food sources of vitamin C include citrus fruits, tomatoes, kiwi, and broccoli. Vitamin E–rich foods include whole grains, nuts, seeds, avocados, and vegetable oils. Selenium, an antioxidant mineral, is found in grains, seeds, and seafood. Foods rich in folate include beans, asparagus, fresh leafy greens, and oranges.

Studies have revealed even more benefits of plant-based foods by demonstrating the dietary effects of plant sterols. Plant stanols and sterols are components that are isolated from the oil of soybeans and of tall pine trees. They are phytochemicals, or chemicals from plants. These are then added as a supplement to certain foods.

Cholesterol is an animal sterol that serves as an integral part of the structure of cell membranes in animals; plant sterols serve the same role in the cell membranes of plants. Because of their structural similarity to cholesterol, plant sterols and stanols will bind with cholesterol during the digestive process. But their subtle differences from cholesterol keep plant sterols from being easily absorbed through the human intestine. Therefore, if a plant sterol binds with cholesterol, it effectively blocks the absorption of that cholesterol through the intestine and promotes its excretion from the body, thus lowering cholesterol levels that circulate in the bloodstream.

Fruits and vegetables not only help your cholesterol profile but also your blood pressure and other contributors to cardiovascular disease. If you add more plant-based foods to your diet, this single beneficial change can have multiple beneficial effects. For maximum nutritional value, choose food with a variety of flavors and colors. Deep, dark leafy greens and bright yellow and orange vegetables are rich in cancer-fighting anti-oxidants as well as essential nutrients.

Whole Grains

Whole grains provide fiber, vitamins, complex carbohydrates, and minerals. Studies show that people who consume more whole grains have a lower risk of heart disease. A whole grain still contains the outer shell, or bran, of the grain and the germ, which would turn into a seedling. Whole grains are superior to processed grains because many nutrients are lost during refining.

When you purchase grain products, look for the terms "whole," "whole wheat," or "whole grain" (not just "wheat") before the name of the grain in the list of ingredients to ensure you are getting the best nutritional value for your money. If you must eat processed grains, choose those that have been enriched, particularly with B vitamins, to replace those nutrients lost during refining.

Diets high in simple carbohydrates (sugar), such as white flours and pasta, can lead to elevated triglyceride levels and reduced levels of HDL or good cholesterol. This increases risks to cardiovascular health and explains why new dietary recommendations emphasize foods high in complex carbohydrates. It's important to note this adverse effect does not occur when the carbohydrates in the diet come from complex carbohydrate sources such as whole grains. These complex carbohydrates, unlike simple carbohydrates, will more slowly release sugar into the bloodstream, causing more steady waves of sugar and insulin, which benefits not only your blood sugar sensitivity but your cholesterol profile as well. Therefore, you should eat whole grains for optimal health and avoid highly refined grains as much as possible.

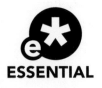

ESSENTIAL

Since grains are rich in fiber and low in fat, they also contribute to a healthy, lower-calorie diet. Most fiber does not get digested and absorbed. Therefore, when you eat the recommended amounts of grains, you feel full without having consumed excess calories. This contrasts greatly with the typical highly processed and refined foods that are quickly digested, high in calories, and do not provide the same feelings of satiety.

Nutrients Found in Whole Foods

When you choose plant-based and whole foods, there are several important nutrients that become part of your diet. These include soluble fiber found in plant-based foods and omega-3 fatty acids.

Soluble Fiber

A huge variety of grains contribute to health, not only as a source of vitamins and minerals but also as a valuable source of complex carbohydrates and soluble fiber. Whole wheat, whole oats, barley, rye, oat bran, rice bran, corn bran, and psyllium seeds all contain soluble fiber. Certain fruits, such as apples, prunes, pears, and oranges, also contain soluble fiber.

Studies show that eating foods that contain soluble fiber can reduce LDL cholesterol levels. In fact, increasing soluble fiber by only 5 to 10g per day is shown to reduce LDL cholesterol by as much as 5 percent. Even more significant reductions in cholesterol levels can be achieved by increasing the daily intake to 10 to 25g per day. Because of this benefit to cholesterol levels, federal government guidelines recommend the use of dietary sources of soluble fiber as a therapeutic option to enhance the reduction of LDL cholesterol for people with high LDL levels.

The reason that soluble fiber helps to lower LDL cholesterol is that it acts much in the same way as prescription bile acid sequestrants. (See Chapter 13 for more information.) In the intestines, soluble fiber binds with cholesterol, making the body unable to absorb it. The cholesterol is then excreted, forcing the liver to dip into its cholesterol reserves to manufacture more bile acids for digestion, resulting in an overall reduction in cholesterol in the body. Insoluble fiber does not have this same cholesterol-binding mechanism, but it does add more bulk to your digested meals that pass through your intestines, reducing your risk of colon cancer. Both types of fiber, since not absorbed in the gut, give a greater feeling of fullness without absorbing as many calories.

Omega-3 Polyunsaturated Fatty Acids

Numerous studies indicate the benefit of increasing foods rich in omega-3 fatty acids in the diet in terms of reducing the risk of heart disease. Deepwater fish such as salmon, tuna, herring, and mackerel are particularly good dietary sources of omega-3 fatty acids. The American Heart

Association guidelines recommend at least two servings of fish per week. Plants can be an excellent source of omega-3 fatty acids as well, including flaxseed, flaxseed oil, and nuts.

Studies show that consumption of foods rich in omega-3 fatty acids offers multiple benefits for heart health. Positive effects include reducing triglyceride levels, reducing risk of sudden death, reducing blood-clotting tendencies, improving blood vessel dilation, and lowering the risk of arrhythmia (irregular heartbeat). Another benefit of consuming fish is that it is a good source of protein that does not contain harmful saturated animal fats. Fish oil also seems to alleviate inflammation and is recommended for people who suffer from joint pain related to arthritis. The reasons these fats produce such beneficial results are unclear.

Eating fish is preferred to consuming fish oil capsules, considering the processing required to convert the fish oil into capsule form; however, concerns exist about high levels of mercury in fish in today's food supply, making filtered and monitored fish oil capsules a viable alternative. Other concerns about carcinogens in farmed fish lead some experts to suggest that wild fish may be more healthful. The debate concerning wild fish, farmed fish, and fish capsules continues, and there are no clear answers yet.

Monounsaturated Vegetable Fats

Research shows that a diet that includes monounsaturated fats reduces total cholesterol and LDL cholesterol levels and has no effect on good cholesterol levels. Nor does consuming foods rich in monounsaturated fats raise triglycerides. This heart-protective effect of monounsaturated fats is believed to partly explain why people who follow a Mediterranean diet that is rich in olive oil live long and healthy lives.

ESSENTIAL

Monounsaturated fats found in plant-based foods can replace saturated fats, according to recommendations endorsed by the American Heart Association. The recommended amount of consumption of these plant-based fats can be up to 20 percent of the total calories in the diet.

Monounsaturated fats are liquid at room temperature and come from vegetables and nuts. Foods that are rich in monounsaturated fats include nuts, avocados, and plant oils such as olive, canola, and peanut.

Polyunsaturated Vegetable Fats

Evidence from research demonstrates that a diet that includes foods rich in polyunsaturated fats, which are even more "unsaturated" than mono-unsaturated fats due to the presence of less calorie-containing hydrogen bonds, reduces LDL cholesterol levels and increases HDL cholesterol levels. Other studies have shown that substituting polyunsaturated fat reduces the risk of heart disease.

Foods that contain polyunsaturated fatty acids include nuts and seeds and also certain plant oils such as corn, safflower, and soybean. Nuts, seeds, and even fish contain polyunsaturated oils. The American Heart Association endorses guidelines to replace saturated fats with polyunsaturated fats up to a total of 10 percent of total calories.

This guideline is important. Just because these fats are healthier does not mean you can consume as much of them as you want. Even the healthiest foods require moderate consumption. Fats are 9 calories per gram, unlike protein and carbohydrates, which are only 4 calories per gram. That means every gram, ounce, or pound of fat you eat has over twice as much weight you can absorb compared with protein or carbohydrates. Eating lots of fats is the fastest way to get fat.

CHAPTER 8

Strategies for Heart-Healthy Eating

Knowing what foods are good for you is only half the story; figuring out how to eat them regularly is the challenging part. Changing your routine is never easy, but you can do it if you keep taking small steady steps. The tips in this chapter will help you to move toward a healthier pattern of eating. Once you start feeling the benefits of enjoying more fresh, wholesome foods, your new habits will become self-reinforcing. Enjoy the process as you travel toward a healthier you.

Eat Healthful Plant-Based Foods

A nutritious diet is key to creating long-term health. Poor nutrition is one of the leading causes of heart disease. The old adage "You are what you eat" is actually quite truthful. Your body derives its nutrients, its building blocks for cellular repair and growth, and its fuel for all activities directly from the food you consume.

The connection between food and your blood-cholesterol levels is direct and powerful. Overconsumption of saturated fats, trans fats, simple sugars, and cholesterol-rich foods leads to overproduction of LDL cholesterol in the liver and to the release of excess amounts of triglycerides into the bloodstream. Saturated fats and cholesterol are present only in animal foods. Trans fats are present only in processed, commercial foods (as described in Chapter 7).

When you alter your eating habits to include more plant-based foods and fewer animal-based and processed foods, you take a powerful step toward improving the health of your bloodstream. Studies have shown that nutritional factors alone can reduce LDL cholesterol by as much as 60 percent in individuals with high levels of cholesterol. This change is far more powerful than the best prescription medications. Another significant difference is that improvements in nutrition do not have the same risk of adverse side effects as taking a long-term prescription drug. In fact, the main side effects of eating healthier are more energy, weight loss, a clearer mind, and more radiant skin. Lastly, eating healthier is much more affordable than medications or other more invasive treatments for heart attack and strokes.

FACT

Based on the amount of efficacy a drug needs to have to be prescribed, if lifestyle changes were a drug, everyone would receive a prescription. In fact, even factoring in the price of whole foods and gym membership, it would be by far the most cost-effective medication ever created.

Numerous nutritional studies demonstrate that plant-based foods enhance your health, particularly cardiovascular health. Humans cannot exist without plant foods. While it is possible to live healthfully over a lifetime without any consumption of meat, it is not possible to survive without eating plant-based foods.

Moving Away from Meats and Animal Fats

Although researchers have determined that a varied diet of whole fresh foods is the most beneficial to health, you can still enjoy meat as part of a heart-healthy diet. You just need to use it carefully. What you need to focus on is creating dishes from lean cuts of meats and enjoying meats as more of a side dish than a main course. Purchase meats from animals fed grass diets, also called "free range," rather than animal fats and animal by-products.

If you eat a typical fast-food diet, it is challenging to convert to a diet of whole fresh foods. The rest of this chapter will provide you with specific strategies for making this transition as smooth as possible. What you eat affects your life in a very intimate way. You need to be able to enjoy your meals and snacks and not feel deprived or punished. Take the time that you need to incorporate healthier foods that you enjoy in order to create lasting changes.

Reducing Saturated Fat in Meats

Eating saturated fats increases the amounts of harmful LDL cholesterol. At the same time, minimizing or avoiding these foods completely in your diet can help to lower harmful LDL cholesterol levels and reduce your risk of heart disease.

When you prepare meats, try to do so in a manner that reduces rather than increases the amount of fat. For example, baste with wines or marinades and season with herbs; grill or broil meats instead of frying or breading; sauté or brown meats in pans sprayed with vegetable oils. If you are adding meat to other dishes, such as spaghetti, brown it first and pour off the fat before you add it to the sauce. Here are some more preparation tips to reduce saturated fats in meats:

- Trim excess fat from meats.
- Purchase lean meats. For beef, aim for 96 percent lean; for chicken, 99 percent lean.
- Avoid purchasing meats that are marbled with fat.
- Remove skin from poultry.
- Broil, grill, roast, or bake meats on racks that allow fats to drain off.
- Skim fat from tops of stews or casseroles.

- Limit or avoid organ meats, such as livers, brains, sweetbreads, and kidneys.
- Limit or avoid processed meats, such as lunchmeat, salami, bologna, pepperoni, or sausage.
- Serve smaller portions of meats.
- Try substituting lean ground turkey or chicken for beef and pork.

These preparation tips will not only reduce the harmful saturated fats in your diet, they will also lower the total fat that you consume, which will help you to manage your weight successfully.

ALERT

Cows are naturally grass-eating animals. Meat from grass-fed cattle has about one-half to one-third the fat as meat from grain-fed cattle. Grass-fed beef is lower in calories and higher in vitamin E, omega-3 fatty acids, and conjugated linoleic acid, another health-enhancing fatty acid.

Lowering Saturated Fats from Dairy Products

While dairy products are a valuable source of calcium and protein, they are not the only sources of these important nutrients. Keep in mind that eating lots of full-fat dairy products increases the levels of saturated fat in your diet, which directly increases your levels of LDL or bad cholesterol. You can still enjoy dairy foods. Simply choose low- or nonfat versions to promote health, and choose milk from dairy cows that have been fed grass diets.

Cheese, in particular, is a very high-fat food, even higher than beef. While you may choose an occasional treat of creamy cheeses, indulging in them regularly will increase your risk of heart disease. Here are some practical tips for lowering the amount of saturated dairy fat in your diet:

- Choose ½ percent, 1 percent, or ideally nonfat milk preferably from grass-fed cows.
- Select nonfat or at least low-fat yogurt, sour cream, and cottage and cream cheese.

- Use lower-fat cheeses for cooking, such as part-skim mozzarella, ricotta, or Parmesan.
- Enjoy rich, creamy, and hard cheeses on special occasions, not daily.
- Limit the use of butter, and use it sparingly.

Check that dairy products come from cows fed grasses and grains rather than meat by-products. Look for other sources of calcium in your diet. Vegetables such as broccoli, chard, greens, and artichokes are all great sources of dietary calcium, as are calcium-fortified orange juice, some whole-grain cereals, and even vitamins. Check the labels.

Avoiding Trans Fats

Keep in mind that there is no level of consumption of trans fats that is not harmful to health. These fats increase your LDL cholesterol and decrease your HDL cholesterol levels. Trans fats are found naturally in some dairy and meat products, but most trans fats in the food supply are created artificially through a process called hydrogenation. This converts a liquid fat to a solid.

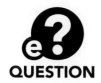

QUESTION

Why do food manufacturers use hydrogenation?
The benefits to food manufacturers of converting vegetable oils to a solid state is that it gives form to otherwise shapeless foods for easier consumption by hand. The process preserves products and extends the shelf life, and it adds flavor.

Trans fats are abundant in processed foods such as cereals, chips, crackers, stick margarine, shortening, lard, and fried fast foods. Remember that trans fats are sometimes manufactured from vegetable oils, so simply because a food manufacturer indicates that something is prepared with vegetable oil does not mean it is trans-fat–free. Also remember that a small "serving" of any food can contain up to 0.49g of trans fat while still reporting 0g on the food label.

When reading food labels on items, look for ingredients such as hydrogenated or partially hydrogenated oils, even if they state 0g of trans fat. If they are listed, try to avoid using these foods. If you must buy a product with such an ingredient, ensure that the hydrogenated ingredient appears at the end of the ingredient list, indicating that it is present in very low quantities. The goal is to live a trans-fat–free life.

You can take the following positive steps to reduce the amounts you consume:

- Avoid or reduce intake of commercially prepared baked goods such as cakes and cookies, snack foods, processed foods, and fast foods.
- Select liquid vegetable oils that contain no trans fats.
- Read margarine labels carefully, and avoid those that contain hydrogenated oils.
- Avoid cooking with lard, shortening, or stick margarine; use vegetable sprays or tub margarine made without trans fats.

ESSENTIAL

For everything that you remove from your diet, you need to introduce something else to replace it. Start by making small changes in your eating habits. Over time, move slowly away from a diet that revolves around animal-based foods, such as meat and dairy products, toward a diet that consists primarily of plant-based foods and fish.

Reduce Intake of Dietary Cholesterol

Dietary cholesterol does not elevate blood-cholesterol levels as much as saturated fat. For most people, excess dietary cholesterol is not an issue. The largest source of dietary cholesterol in America is eggs. Studies show that in healthy individuals, consuming one egg per day did not lead to elevated cholesterol levels. If, however, you think that you may be overeating cholesterol, here are some tips on how to reduce your dietary intake:

- Eat egg whites instead of whole eggs.
- Purchase eggs from chickens raised on a vegetarian diet rather than animal fats and animal by-products.

- Read egg carton labels and compare brands to purchase the most nutritious eggs.
- Limit intake of shellfish high in cholesterol, such as shrimp, abalone, crayfish, and squid. (Other forms of shellfish are not excessively high in cholesterol and can provide valuable nutrients.)

Increasing Vegetables and Fruits

As you reduce the amount of meat you consume, gradually increase the amount of vegetables in your diet. Over time, your taste buds will evolve, and you will enjoy more of the subtle flavors of vegetables and fruits. Your meals will be equally tasty but more colorful and will include more fiber and plant-based nutrients. This reduces not only your risk of cardiovascular disease, but also for diabetes and certain types of cancer.

Try to incorporate fruits or vegetables in every meal and as snacks. Reduce the amount of meat or chicken in typical combination dishes. For example, in spaghetti, reduce the amount of beef or substitute ground turkey. Then increase the vegetable content in your sauces by adding more mushrooms, green peppers, celery, and carrots.

Here are some more tips on how to include more vegetables in your daily diet:

- At breakfast, slice half a banana or toss some berries or raisins on your cereal.
- Add frozen fruits such as berries or peaches to hot cereals.
- At meals, serve larger portions of vegetables, or prepare multiple vegetable dishes and have meat as a side dish.
- Prepare meats with fruit toppings or marinades instead of butter.
- Enjoy fruit-based desserts such as poached pears, baked apples, or fresh-fruit sorbets.
- Buy packaged, prewashed, and sliced veggies to pack as snacks.
- Eat fresh whole fruits that are in season as snacks with meals or between them.
- Add legumes such as peas or beans into rice or pasta dishes.
- Incorporate multiple vegetables into salads in addition to lettuce.
- Enjoy a smoothie made with fruits or vegetables as a beverage.

Keep in mind that all these fruits and vegetables add up to less weight, less disease, less disability, more energy, and a healthy, glowing appearance.

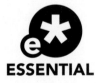

ESSENTIAL

Fruits and vegetables are a great source of fiber. Soluble fiber that's part of a healthy diet can reduce blood-cholesterol levels and the amount of calories you absorb. Some fruits and vegetables that contain soluble fiber, in addition to numerous other beneficial nutrients, include apples with peels, oranges, figs, prunes, peas, broccoli, and carrots.

Enjoying Whole Grains

Whole-grain foods are minimally processed and therefore rich in vitamins, minerals, and fiber. Grains include whole wheat, brown rice, barley, rye, oatmeal, and corn. Whole grains provide complex carbohydrates that are essential for energy and vitamins A and E, magnesium, calcium, and other important nutrients. These fiber-rich foods contain both soluble and insoluble fiber, but they mostly contain insoluble fiber, which aids digestion, keeps your colon healthy, and makes you feel full, helping with weight management. Processed grains, in contrast, are simple carbohydrates and have lost many of the nutrients and the fiber.

Oatmeal that contains oat bran is a rich source of soluble fiber that can help to lower cholesterol levels. Food manufacturers often remove the oat bran in the instant-cook varieties. Be sure to purchase whole oats or oat bran to obtain the cholesterol-lowering results.

Ideally, you should eat six servings of grains per day. Here are some tips to add more whole grains into your daily diet:

- Include a grain-based food at every meal.
- Make sure the food is labeled "whole" on the front and in the ingredients list.
- Try whole-grain rolls, breadsticks, crackers, and muffins for snacks.
- Prepare desserts with fruits and whole grains, such as apple crisp.
- Sprinkle wheat germ into your cereals or smoothies.

- Use whole-grain tortillas or pita breads to make healthy chips for dips or salsas.
- Use whole-grain pasta, whole-grain bread for sandwiches, and even whole-grain pizza bread.

FACT

Whole oats are a rich source of soluble fiber. Studies show that consuming 10 to 25g of soluble fiber per day can lower cholesterol by 10 percent. Portions that contain as little as 5 to 10g of soluble fiber can lower LDL cholesterol by as much as 5 percent. Three-quarters of a cup of uncooked oatmeal or half a cup of oat bran contains 3g of soluble fiber.

Increasing Good Fats—Vegetable Oils, Nuts, and Fish

Research shows that the types of fats you eat strongly affect your cholesterol levels. While saturated and trans fats increase your LDL or bad cholesterol, unsaturated fats (including monounsaturated fats and polyunsaturated fats) actually reduce levels of bad cholesterol and increase levels of good cholesterol. Unsaturated fats are found in plant-based products such as most vegetable oils, nuts, seeds, and whole grains. The one nonplant source of these good fats is deepwater or fatty fish, which is a rich source of polyunsaturated fat.

Dietary fat is not the "enemy." Heart-protective unsaturated fats play an important part in a healthy diet. The key is to try to watch what type of fat you eat—reduce saturated fats, eliminate trans fats, and then replace those fats with unsaturated fats in the diet. This does not give you permission to consume as much fat as you want as long as it is "healthy fat." Remember, every gram of fat has over twice as many calories as a gram of protein or calories. To maintain a healthy weight, you still want to eat only a small portion of healthy fats. Here are some tips on how to incorporate unsaturated fats into your daily diet:

- Cook with unsaturated liquid vegetable oils such as canola, safflower, grape seed, or ideally olive oil, which has shown to have the most benefits.
- If you must use some sort of butter or margarine, buy tub or liquid margarines with an unsaturated vegetable oil, such as soybean oil, as the first ingredient.
- Throw a few nuts or sesame seeds into your morning cereal. Foods that contain monounsaturated fats include almonds, cashews, peanuts, and walnuts.
- Spread natural peanut butter on celery sticks or green peppers for a healthy snack.
- Dip bread in limited amounts of olive oil instead of spreading on butter.
- Enjoy deepwater fish on occasion.
- Use flax seeds or powder as a topping or ingredient in grain dishes.

Omega-3 Fatty Acids

Another important heart-health benefit is found in polyunsaturated fats that include omega-3 (linolenic) and omega-6 (linoleic) fatty acids. Researchers have found that omega-3 fatty acids have an anti-inflammatory effect. They also reduce the likelihood of forming blood clots, help blood vessels to relax or dilate, and can lower levels of LDL cholesterol. The primary source of omega-3 fatty acids is fish. Fish that come from cold, deep water are the best source of omega-3s. The American Heart Association recommends eating fatty fish at least twice a week. More recent information, however, about high mercury levels in fish and high carcinogen levels in farmed fish has caused concern, so be careful about the fish you buy. Like anything else, moderation of fish consumption likely offers some of the benefits of omega-3 fatty acids while minimizing the risk of fish consumption.

Flaxseed and Flaxseed Oil

Flaxseed also contains high levels of omega-3 fatty acids and does not present the same mercury or carcinogenic concerns as fish. Using flaxseed, however, requires some care. Flaxseed must be ground up in order for the body to absorb the oils, and it cannot be cooked as heat will destroy the oils.

ESSENTIAL

You can also take fish oil supplements. A dose of about 4g of fish oil is considered beneficial. Finding high-quality supplements, however, is always a concern. Search for those from highly reputable producers that affirm that the oils have been filtered for toxins such as mercury.

If you decide to add flaxseed into your diet, grind the seeds before you eat them. You can sprinkle ground flaxseed on cereal. Remember to store flaxseed in the refrigerator so the oil does not go rancid. If you purchase flaxseed oil, you can use it in salad dressings or on pasta, but do not cook with it. Based on results from research studies, the best amount to consume to achieve cholesterol-lowering results is 50g per day. Any amount is likely beneficial, though.

Raise a Glass to the Benefits of Moderate Drinking

Excessive drinking of alcohol is never a good practice. Heavy drinking can lead to high blood pressure and heart rhythm problems, as well as liver damage. For women, studies show that alcohol intake increases the risk of breast cancer. According to government statistics, up to 10 percent of U.S. adults misuse alcohol. Abstention from alcohol is the best practice for people who cannot enjoy it in moderation.

For those who can enjoy alcoholic beverages in moderation, however, studies show that alcohol consumption is associated with a lower risk of death from heart disease. Scientists have not identified the precise reasons why low amounts of alcohol consumption may reduce the risk of heart disease. Some experts theorize that it may be because it increases HDL cholesterol. Furthermore, the benefits occur regardless of which alcoholic beverage is consumed, meaning it is simply the ethanol in the alcohol that provides the positive results. Though low amounts of alcohol reduce cardiovascular risk, alcohol can increase the risk for many other diseases. Alcohol consumption comes with an increased risk of liver disease, gastritis, pancreatic disease, cancer, and many more diseases. These risks certainly outweigh any benefits in those who drink a significant amount of alcohol.

FACT

One drink is equal to five ounces of wine, twelve ounces of beer, or an ounce and a half of eighty-proof whiskey. For heart-health benefits, consume drinks with meals. No one should begin drinking alcoholic beverages if they do not already drink alcohol.

For wine enthusiasts, the news is even better. In addition to the HDL-raising benefits of alcohol, red wine also contains phytochemicals. These are plant-based chemicals that provide health benefits when consumed. The grape skins used in making red wine are full of compounds known as flavonoids. Flavonoids are known to help prevent LDL cholesterol from oxidizing and turning into the kind of early plaque that may adhere to arterial walls. Flavonoids also prevent blood clots, further reducing risk of a heart attack or stroke.

Regardless of any cardiovascular benefit, no one should ever increase alcohol consumption to, in theory, improve his health. While it may provide some cardiovascular benefit, this benefit comes with other risks. Generally, those who drink socially may have their cardiovascular profile improved somewhat, while anyone who drinks as often as daily should consider cutting down.

How to Read Food Labels

Eating right can help you to feel better, have more energy, manage your weight more effectively, and help you to live a longer life with less risk of disability and disease. You know that you want to decrease the saturated fats, trans fats, and simple sugars in your diet and increase the mono- and poly-unsaturated fats, whole foods, and complex carbohydrates. But where do you begin? First, you need to understand how to read food labels. Next, you need some tips for navigating the aisles of your favorite grocery store.

What to Look For

The U.S. Food and Drug Administration regulates food labels. Labels must include not only a list of nutrients but also a list of ingredients. These are both sources of valuable information. In the nutrient list, the important items to check include the total fats and the breakdown of the types of fats included, as well as the total carbohydrates and breakdown of fiber and sugar.

Aim for approximately 300 to 350g of complex carbohydrates, of which at least 20 to 30g are fiber. Also aim for at least 60g of lean protein daily, though you may need more if younger or an athlete. With fat, try to limit consumption to a maximum of 60g daily but aim for less. Make sure to maximize unsaturated fat and minimize saturated and trans fat.

In the total fat section, check to see how much saturated fat and total fat are listed. Remember, "bad" fats that you should limit or avoid are saturated fat, trans fat, and—to a limited extent—cholesterol. "Good" fats that you can include are monounsaturated and polyunsaturated fats.

In the carbohydrate section of the label, check how much dietary fiber and sugar are in the product. Select foods that are higher in dietary fiber and as low as possible in sugar. When making a buying decision, compare products to find those that contain good fats instead of bad fats and that are high in fiber and whole grains.

Understanding the List of Ingredients

The ingredient list also provides a wealth of valuable information. Ingredients are listed in order of magnitude, with the items used in larger amounts listed first and smallest amounts at the end. Try to choose foods that feature grains, lean proteins, and fruits and vegetables at the start of the list, and have the fat and oil ingredients toward the end of the list.

Choose products that list the specific type of vegetable oil—olive oil, for example—rather than labels that use a generic "vegetable oil" listing. Often when manufacturers use the term "vegetable oil," the product includes tropical oils such as palm or coconut that contain saturated fats, rather than the healthier monounsaturated and polyunsaturated fats. To avoid trans fats, stay away from products that list hydrogenated or partially hydrogenated vegetable oils.

When it comes to grain products, choose products with the words "whole," "whole wheat," or "whole grain" in front of the grain ingredient, as well as terms like "bran" or "germ." Sometimes food manufacturers will use enriched flour and dye it a brown color to make it appear like a whole grain. If the ingredient list shows enriched flour as the main ingredient, the grains are highly processed, even if it is enriched "wheat" flour. These are not whole grains, and the product is likely to be high in sugar and low in fiber. Read carefully.

Take Your Time

Be prepared to spend a little more time on your grocery shopping to allow you to read labels. However, once you have selected foods you like that prominently feature healthful ingredients, you can return to your faster style of moving through aisles and throwing items in your shopping basket. As you work your way through the fine print on labels, keep in mind that you are what you eat. This task of careful shopping, while tedious and time-consuming at first, will pay great dividends to your better health in the long run and ultimately will become fairly quick and easy.

Your Shopping List

An important strategy that can go a long way toward improving your food choices is to prepare a shopping list before you go to the store. This helps you to resist the newest, flashiest, and trendiest food products that are designed to catch your eye.

Note that the outer edges of the store tend to have the healthiest foods. These include the fresh fruits and vegetables, meats, breads, and dairy products. The inner aisles are filled with processed foods and ready-to-eat preparations that are full of saturated and trans fats, sugar, and salt. Remember that you want to select a balance of foods from each of the food groups.

From the bread and cereal group, choose whole-grain products like breads and muffins. You can also buy whole-grain pita bread, tortillas, pasta, and rice cakes. Choose whole-grain flour for baking and items such as brown or wild rice and whole corn or flour tortillas. Select whole-grain, unsweetened cereals or whole-grain hot cereals like oatmeal.

ESSENTIAL

As a careful shopper, over time you may become familiar with the manufacturers that create the healthier foods you want. You can gravitate toward those brands with more assurance that you are selecting items that will both taste good and be good for you. When purchasing something for the first time, it is still a good idea to check out the ingredients, no matter who the manufacturer.

From the fruit and vegetable group, select a variety of fresh foods. Today's frozen and canned vegetables can have as much nutritional value as fresh vegetables. If you're busy, you may have concerns that stocking up on fresh fruits and vegetables is wasteful. Go ahead and buy frozen products. If you buy canned vegetables, either go with a low-sodium variety or rinse the vegetables before serving. Canned fruits should come packed in juice, not syrup.

Another time-saver are packaged, prewashed, presliced vegetables. These are ideal for snacks and salads. They may cost slightly more, but if they help you to incorporate more vegetables into your diet, you will save more in the long run from your health dividends as you age. Fruit and vegetable juices are also good selections, especially if you can find fresh juices. Also be sure the fruit juice you buy is either 100 percent fruit juice or juice and water with no added sugar.

When choosing dairy and meat, remember the guidelines you learned earlier in this chapter. Look for low- or nonfat milk, cheese, and yogurt and lean cuts of meat. You can also select alternative sources of protein such as beans, nuts, and lentils.

Meal Planning for Health

Maintaining healthy nutrition does require some planning. However, with a minimal amount of organization, you can keep health-enhancing foods in your refrigerator and cupboards. Now let's look at how you can use these tips to plan healthy meals. Incorporate even a handful of these suggestions into your daily life, and before you realize it, you will have shifted to a healthier overall eating pattern. Each of these changes becomes easier with time and eventually can become automatic.

Which types of cooking oils should I buy?
Choose either monounsaturated vegetable oils, which include olive, canola, peanut, avocado, almond, hazelnut, and pecan, or polyunsaturated vegetable oils, such as corn, safflower, sunflower, sesame, soybean, and cottonseed.

Breakfast

Breakfast is the most important meal of the day because it ends the long period of body starvation, otherwise known as sleep. That is how breakfast earned its name: You are "breaking the fast." It's also a wonderful opportunity to eat fiber-rich foods. Plan to include a combination of fiber-rich and protein-rich foods, along with either a fruit or vegetable serving. Great sources of fiber for breakfast include hot or cold whole grain cereals and breads. Breakfast protein can come from nonfat or low-fat dairy products such as milk. You can add fruits or vegetables either by drinking one glass of juice or by mixing fruit with your cereal dish or having it on the side. Another great breakfast option is a smoothie. These are easy to make in a blender, with or without low-fat milk, some fruits, and wheat germ or ground flaxseed. All of these options can help you start your day on the right foot.

Lunch

Lunch is another great opportunity for a rich source of fiber and more fruits and vegetables. Try sandwiches on hearty whole-grain breads with fresh tomatoes, lettuce, and sprouts. You can also try using whole-grain pitas, tortillas, or wraps. You may prefer whole-grain pasta. For vegetable sources of protein, use bean dips such as hummus on a sandwich or nuts on the side.

If packing a lunch, include a vegetable and some fruit. For example, take some prewashed, prepackaged baby carrots or celery sticks. Or slice up a bell pepper into sticks. Easily portable fruits include apples, bananas, oranges, nectarines, grapes, and pears. There are also numerous types of prepackaged sliced fruits for your convenience. Try to eat fruits that are fresh and in season.

Salads are a great lunch that can be made more filling by adding beans or starches such as whole-grain pastas. Soups are a fantastic source of multiple vegetables and beans, but watch your salt intake as that can raise blood pressure. If you combine soups or salads with some hearty whole-grain breads or muffins, you can have a satisfying and nutrient-packed meal. For dessert, try some fresh fruit or poached, baked, or frozen fruits, such as poached pears, baked apples, or fresh fruit sorbets.

FACT

Simple sugars are not "bad" in and of themselves, but when consumed in excess, they can have a harmful effect on cholesterol levels. Studies show that a diet high in simple sugars, which includes refined carbohydrates (enriched-flour breads and pastas) and hard candy, actually increases triglyceride levels and decreases levels of HDL or good cholesterol, in addition to promoting insulin resistance, an early form of diabetes.

Dinner

For dinner, try to shift the emphasis to a vegetable- and grain-based main course with any meat dishes on the side. Or, in meals that call for sauces, use a combination of vegetables and meats to reduce the total amount of meat that you consume. For example, you can cut the amount of meat in stew in half and instead add in extra carrots, celery, and mushrooms. You can try chili with beans and no meat, or use ground turkey instead of beef and add more vegetables instead of meats. Try enjoying stir-fried vegetable dishes with only a small amount of skinless chicken, or simply use tofu instead of any meat product.

Keep in mind that when you eat beans, peas, or lentils together with a dairy product or with grains such as bread or rice, you can obtain the same amount of protein from your meal as if you had consumed a meat dish. Other benefits of eating more beans instead of meat is that they are much more affordable, they contain no saturated fats and no cholesterol, they are nutrient dense, and they are valuable sources of dietary fiber.

If you use canned beans in your foods, try to buy low-sodium varieties and use the liquid that they come packed in for cooking. That liquid is rich in soluble fiber—that's why it has that thick consistency.

Heart-Healthy Dining for Winning Results

Dietary changes are very powerful. Blood-cholesterol levels show signs of improvement in as few as three to four weeks. Over several months, LDL levels can be reduced through dietary changes by as much as 60 percent! This reduces the risk of suffering a debilitating or deadly heart attack or stroke.

Keep in mind, however, that you must make a lifestyle change toward a healthier pattern of eating and not treat this as a short-term, fad diet for quick and easy weight loss. Eating healthy for life represents a commitment—to yourself and to those you love—to make a daily difference in supporting health through the foods that you eat. Treats are definitely a part of that picture. But for the most part, your daily diet will be one that is full of nutrient-dense, health-enhancing foods for a longer, healthier, and more enjoyable life.

Read the heart-healthy recipes in Chapters 16, 17, 18, and 19 for more ideas on how to plan tasty, enjoyable, and nutritious meals for your entire family's health and pleasure. These recipes, from the National Heart, Lung, and Blood Institute, were developed under the direction of leading medical and nutritional scientists during government-sponsored research and education projects devoted to keeping Americans healthy. These recipes have been specifically designed and tested to promote health. Now you can use the results of this important research to improve your personal health.

This collection includes a variety of ethnic dishes to find something to please every taste. Even children love these recipes. In addition, each recipe includes a nutrient breakdown so you know exactly what you're eating. Remember, heart-healthy cooking does not mean a sacrifice of flavor or pleasure.

CHAPTER 9

Successful Weight Management

Healthy weight management is an important part of a healthy lifestyle. Maintaining a healthy weight requires understanding what causes weight gain and the key strategies to prevent it, as you will learn in this chapter. A healthy weight requires a combination of good nutrition, consistent physical activity, and effective stress management, which are important factors of a healthy cholesterol profile as well. When you keep your weight at a healthy level, you will live longer with more energy and fewer disabilities.

What Is a Healthy Weight?

A healthy weight is one that minimizes your risk of illness and disease and falls within the range of weight appropriate for your height. A person may suffer from poor health if overly heavy. Similarly, a person can experience poor health if overly thin. Therefore, a reasonable weight goal is in between those two extremes. Among individuals this can fall within a broad range, as people come in a variety of sizes and shapes due to strong genetic factors. Each person should find his own healthy weight for his own body type.

Understanding Body Composition

It's not just the size of the package that is important, it's what is inside the package that counts. Your body is composed of fat mass and lean body mass. Together, this is referred to as your body composition. Ideally, you want to keep the percentage of fat quite a bit lower than the percentage of nonfat mass. (Your nonfat mass includes your bones, organs, and muscle.) And, if you decide to lose weight, you want to lose fat, not valuable muscle tissue that gives you strength and support.

FACT

The good news for those who are overweight is that even a small reduction in weight, as little as 10 percent of total body weight, leads to remarkable improvements in health. For example, research subjects who lost 10 percent of total body weight have experienced reductions in high blood pressure, blood glucose, and bad cholesterol levels, as well as improvements in body composition. Those who lose weight have a tremendous reduction of disease.

Just because a person appears to be thin does not make him healthy. Some people who are thin in appearance are actually unhealthy when it comes to body composition. Typically, they are weak, sedentary, and may be smokers. They may eat very little food and have an unbalanced diet. Oftentimes, people with this type of profile believe they are healthy as long as they are thin. They could not be more mistaken.

Being significantly underweight poses serious threats to good health. For premenopausal women, being too underweight can lead to infertility or osteoporosis. People who suffer from disorders such as anorexia or bulimia also experience poor health. In particular, people who are anorectic will consume muscle tissue from their body's stores to survive when fat stores are depleted, including tissue from the heart muscle. It is not uncommon for people who are recovering from anorexia to have a heart attack when the weight they begin to gain creates excess stress on an already weakened heart.

At the same time, a person who may be more stocky and robust in appearance but who exercises regularly, eats a balanced diet of nutrient-rich fresh foods, and who does not smoke, is much healthier.

The message, therefore, is not that thin is in or that every person must have the same body. Rather, the message is that you should aim to maintain a weight that is healthy for you and your body type.

All Body Fat Is Not Equal

To make matters even more complex, researchers have found that the amount of body fat is not the only factor that is important. What is equally (if not more) significant is where the fat is deposited on your body. Studies show that people whose bodies store fat around the abdominal area, also referred to as an "apple shaped" body, are at higher risk of heart disease, stroke, high blood pressure, and Type 2 diabetes than those people who are more "pear shaped" and carry their excess fat around their legs and thighs. Unfortunately, it's hard to dictate where your fat goes, but you can dictate how much of it you have.

QUESTION

Why does abdominal fat create a higher risk of heart disease than fat elsewhere?
The exact reasons why abdominal fat poses greater risks are not known, but one factor may be that abdominal fat puts greater stress on internal organs that become surrounded with fat.

To determine whether you have abdominal obesity, you need to measure your waist circumference. For purposes of this measurement, your waist is considered to be halfway between the lowest rib and the top of your hipbone, measured when you are upright and your trunk is perpendicular to the floor. A waist circumference of greater than forty inches for men, or greater than thirty-five inches for women, may indicate a higher risk of heart disease. Abdominal obesity is also considered one of the risk factors of the metabolic syndrome (see Chapter 14).

The Body Mass Index

Another method to assess whether your weight may put you at risk is to calculate your body mass index (BMI). The BMI expresses weight relative to height. It provides a general guideline to check whether you are in a healthy weight range. A high BMI score may indicate increased risks for heart disease, high blood pressure, diabetes, and high cholesterol. BMI guidelines are not accurate for estimating risks for people who are healthy at higher weight levels, such as muscular competitive athletes or pregnant women. These guidelines also do not apply to growing children or frail and sedentary older adults.

Instructions for calculating your BMI are included in Appendix B. If your BMI is greater than 25, you fall into the category of being overweight. A BMI between 18.5 and 24.9 is considered a healthy weight. If your BMI score is less than 18.5, you are considered to be underweight.

Beyond Your Looks

Losing excess fat is not only an important factor in reducing the risk of cardiovascular disease but also in reducing the risk of many diseases, including gallbladder disease, diabetes, and cancer.

In addition to the reduced risk for numerous diseases, losing weight provides multiple physical, mental, and emotional benefits. People who lose excess fat weight feel better, have more energy, have fewer aches and pains, and can enjoy a higher quality of life. People may also experience an improved sense of self-esteem and a feeling of greater control over their life that leads to a greater sense of self-confidence.

Excess weight strains your heart and your circulatory system. Your heart must work harder to pump more blood through your body, causing higher blood pressure. Extra weight also strains your musculoskeletal system and puts greater stress on your joints, increasing arthritis and back pain.

People who carry excess weight are more likely to have certain risk factors for cardiovascular disease, including high LDL cholesterol, low HDL cholesterol, high triglycerides, Type 2 diabetes, or high blood pressure. At the same time, when people who are overweight lose excess body fat, even as few as five to ten pounds, they can typically expect reductions in their total cholesterol, LDL cholesterol, and triglycerides, accompanied by increases in HDL cholesterol. All of these benefits combined are much greater than the sum of their parts.

FACT

More than 60 percent of adults in the United States are overweight or obese. Being overweight can contribute to high LDL cholesterol, low HDL cholesterol, high VLDL cholesterol, and high triglycerides, all of which increase risk for cardiovascular disease.

Causes of Weight Gain

In simplistic terms, one can say that the cause of weight gain is taking in excess calories. But this does not take into full consideration the complex social factors that make it difficult to live an active lifestyle, to enjoy wholesome fresh foods, and to separate emotional factors from the need to eat. Furthermore, as researchers learn more and more about the differences among people's metabolic profiles, it seems that depending on what types of foods are consumed, some people are more prone to gain weight easily and to have a more difficult time losing it. The overall picture is complex, but a few simple factors play key roles.

Supersizing of Foods

In this day and age, it is easy for people to overeat. The supersizing of food portions by food manufacturers adds to this tendency. Since most of the cost of food production is in the labor and not in the raw materials, food producers have financial incentives to increase the size of food products in order to attract more customers. The increased amount of cost involved in providing a larger serving size is outweighed by the greater number of customers who purchase their product, since it is perceived as a better value or more food for the money. This perception of value by consumers, however, fails to take into consideration that they are actually purchasing more food than they need. And all that excess consumption leads to excess weight. Consumers might think they are paying just a little bit more for a lot more food, but in actuality they are paying much more for the harm the extra food does to their bodies.

In fact, this issue is so prevalent that the U.S. Federal Trade Commission and more recently the U.S. Food and Drug Administration recommended that manufacturers reexamine the portion sizes on food labels. The FTC and FDA have made this recommendation based on the fact that "they [food labels] may significantly understate the amount of particular foods and calories that people typically consume."

Officials at the FTC believe that current food-labeling practices confuse consumers over serving sizes so that consumers "may underestimate the number of calories and other nutrients that they eat." For example, a typical three-ounce bag of chips is labeled as "two servings" but packaged as a single serving. Twenty-ounce soft drinks are also packaged as a single serving but described as two servings on the food label. The FTC recommends that the FDA look at whether serving-size listings are "sufficiently clear and prominent."

Until government officials clear up current labeling practices, however, it is up to you to make judgments about serving sizes on your own. Generally, serving sizes are much smaller than typical portion sizes, so you consume more fat, carbohydrates, and calories than are listed for a single serving. To get a better idea of how much you consume, you must try to determine the number of servings you are eating by paying attention to the serving size as compared to your portion size. Take time to read food labels carefully, and compare the weight of the package with what is noted as the weight of a serving on the label. Also, read the serving-size guidelines at the end of this chapter carefully.

Emotional Overeating

While emotional overeating may not rise to the level of a clinical eating disorder, many people overeat in response to cues that are completely unrelated to hunger. Stress can play a role, as can environmental factors in the home. For example, if your parents rewarded you with a food treat when you accomplished tasks, you may continue to give yourself this type of treat when you finish something as an adult. Similarly, if food was used to cope with emotions rather than discussing, facing, or experiencing them, it can continue to play that role in adult life.

ESSENTIAL

Researchers suggest that if you eat the foods you really like in measured amounts with meals and avoid them when you are hungry, you can reduce your cravings. The reason is that by giving in to your body's desire for certain foods, you train your body to want that treat even more. For example, if you only eat chocolate when you're ravenous, you increase the strength of your cravings.

Keeping a journal can be helpful for people who find that they eat in response to these types of emotional cues rather than because they are experiencing true feelings of hunger. In the journal, you can record what triggered an eating episode, what you were thinking and feeling at the time, and what feelings you were avoiding by eating. This process may be very revealing as you start to unravel some of your more unconscious eating behaviors that lead to overconsumption of food.

Eating Highly Refined, Processed Foods

Another factor that can contribute to overeating is choosing foods that are highly refined and processed. In this case, the overeating often occurs in response to genuine hunger cues. For example, breads and pastas that are made with enriched flour rather than with whole grains lack fiber that provides important feelings of fullness and satiety. Drinking juices instead of eating fruits is also another missed opportunity to eat fiber-rich foods.

Fiber, both soluble and insoluble, is critically important to health. Not only does it provide roughage that is good for digestion, but it also lowers cholesterol levels and makes you feel full. It truly is hard to overeat when your meals are filled with wholesome fresh fruits, vegetables, and whole grains that have bulk and are steadily absorbed.

Lack of Physical Activity

Living an active lifestyle in today's technology-driven world is a challenge. It is actually much easier to live a sedentary life today than it is to live an active life. Many people start their day by traveling to work or to school via cars or buses. They spend much of their day seated in chairs with few breaks from their sitting lifestyle. When they return home at the end of the day, they are tired and hungry and the last thing they feel like doing is "exercising."

FACT

All day long, you use devices that remove movement from your day. You drive a car, take escalators and elevators, use automatic door and garage openers, and have remote controls for every form of device. You shop, perform research, play games, and communicate with others via your computer. You order food delivered to your home.

Without a conscious effort to move, it's actually quite easy to remain inactive all day long. When this lack of movement is combined with over-consumption of foods, it's easy to see how the combination can quickly add to increased weight gain.

Loss of Lean Body Mass

An aspect of the picture that affects metabolism and activity levels is the natural decline in lean body mass that occurs with aging. After the age of thirty-five, both men and women lose approximately one-third to one-half pound of muscle each year. If your total weight is not changing, this means that this loss of lean body mass has been replaced by an equivalent gain of fat mass. Although your weight may not have changed, the difference between these two types of tissues is extremely significant from the standpoint of weight management.

The loss of lean body mass means your body is composed of less of the metabolically more active tissue as well as a decrease in the muscle that provides strength to move and accomplish physical tasks. So not only is the body burning fewer calories even at rest, but it also becomes more tired and less capable of doing things such as walking up the stairs, running after children, and lifting and carrying grocery bags.

ESSENTIAL

Health benefits can be gained from even a modest weight loss. You do not need to become a size two or look like a cover model. You just need to be sure that you lose the weight in a healthy way. As with cholesterol, blood pressure, blood sugar, and smoking, even small changes in your weight can go a long way.

This is the beginning of a cycle of reduced daily physical activity that leads to even more fat gain. Over time, the ratio of fat becomes high and the amount of lean is low. The older adult may no longer have the strength even to climb a flight of stairs or get up and move around at all, and the pounds can easily add up. Basically, the less you move, the less muscle you have and more weight you gain, so the less you want to move. The key is to interrupt and turn around this vicious cycle. The more you move, the slimmer you will be. You'll have more muscle and energy, motivating you to keep moving.

Why Dieting Does Not Work

Diets that involve simply avoiding food altogether, known as starvation diets, don't work. You need to eat nutritious foods to lose weight and keep it down. When you starve yourself, you lose both fat and hard-earned muscle tissue. This loss of lean body mass from dieting results in a decreased resting metabolic rate, similar to when people lose lean body mass as they age. Therefore, just starving yourself will slow your metabolism down, yet you will eventually eat more due to your hunger, now with a slower metabolism to burn less of what you eat. In the long run, you will do more harm than good and gain more weight than you lose. That is why starvation diets have a nearly 100 percent failure rate. This cycle of weight loss and gain is called the yo-yo effect.

ALERT

If you're out of shape, a new regular exercise program can build up your muscles. It may seem discouraging at first because you may see a weight gain. (Remember, muscle weighs more than fat.) But for every pound of muscle you gain, you also burn about thirty to fifty more calories a day, for the same amount of effort. Over time, the added muscle will help you lose and manage your weight.

"Yo-yo" dieting is the tendency for people to lose and regain the same weight over and over again, rather than make any permanent changes in weight management. Some researchers believe that this is even more detrimental to health than not dieting at all.

Healthy weight loss should occur at the rate of no more than one to two pounds per week. At this healthy rate, you are losing body fat rather than muscle tissue. You are also more likely to keep it off and avoid the yo-yo syndrome.

What Does Work

The bottom line when it comes to weight management is that lifestyle changes will help to bring your weight to a healthy level. Depending on how much excess fat you have, this process may take a longer time. However, any lifestyle changes you are able to make will improve your health and your feelings of well-being.

Do Your Best to Be Your Best

Managing your weight is part of a healthy lifestyle. To achieve success, it's best to make changes gradually and to have realistic expectations. The following tips can help you get started:

- Examine your eating habits. Are you meeting the necessary requirements?
- Portion size matters. Learn what healthy single servings of food are, and adjust your portion sizes.
- Get active each and every day. Every movement counts.
- Incorporate strength or weight training to increase your lean body mass.

As you improve your daily habits, instead of focusing on changes in your scale weight, notice changes in how you feel. Do you have more energy? Are you feeling stronger? Are you sleeping better at night?

If you're the type who needs a goal in the form of a number, such as weight, to keep you motivated, think about measuring your progress in other ways. Get your cholesterol and blood-sugar levels tested. Check whether your resting heart rate and blood pressure levels are going down. Most important, know you're doing the best that you can for your long-term well-being.

ESSENTIAL

The best approach for weight management is one that is grounded in the following basics: healthy nutrition, regular physical activity that includes lifestyle activity, and stress management. For details on how to incorporate these healthy lifestyle habits into your life, see the chapter that treats the specific topic (Chapters 8, 10, and 11, respectively).

Avoid Overeating

While it is important to eat a diet full of foods that enhance health and to avoid eating those foods that can be harmful to health, keep in mind that overeating any foods can lead to excess weight that is harmful to health. One of the ways to avoid overeating is to learn what a reasonable serving size should look like. Here are some helpful visual cues:

- One serving of fresh fruit or vegetables is about the size of a tennis ball.
- One serving of canned fruit or cooked vegetables is about the size of a computer mouse.

- One serving of dried fruit is about the size of a golf ball.
- One serving of fruit as juice measures ¾ cup.*
- One serving of vegetable juice measures 1 cup.*
- One serving of sliced bread is about the width of a centimeter.
- One serving of cold cereal is about the size of a baseball.
- One serving of hot cereal is about the size of an English muffin.
- One serving of rice or pasta is about the size of a regular scoop of ice cream.

*It is recommended that as many of your servings as possible come from whole fruit and vegetables, with no more than half of your fruit and vegetable servings be from fruit juice since juice does not provide the same amount of dietary fiber as the fruit itself.

Restaurants tend to promote overeating, with large portions laden with oil and fat and the encouragement of appetizers, sides, and desserts. In addition, most restaurants do not list their ingredients or nutritional information, leaving you ignorant of their food's contents. There are several strategies you can use to avoid overeating when you are eating out. For instance, you can share a main course with a friend, order a meal of various side dishes, or simply take half of the order home to eat later. Also, more and more restaurants have a healthier or "guilt-free" menu, typically meals with more vegetables and grilled lean meats as opposed to fried foods. If you have the opportunity to plan ahead, often restaurants will list the nutritional information for their menu on their website. Occasionally, you can get a copy of the menu's nutritional information on request.

Another way to avoid overeating is to eat the recommended amounts of grains, fruits, and vegetables. The high fiber content of these foods help you to feel satiated, and when you are feeling so full, you are much less likely to overeat.

Keep in mind that lifestyle habits are not easy to change. Be gentle with yourself and appreciate your small successes on a daily basis. Over time, you will find that your life has transformed in so many more ways than simply managing your weight. The weight that you lose, whatever the amount, represents your body's quest to find its best balance in the midst of a lifestyle dedicated to creating health.

CHAPTER 10

Getting Active

Along with eating a balanced diet of minimally processed whole foods, being active on most days of the week is critical to creating healthy cholesterol levels. Getting active for health does not mean spending hours at the gym. In fact, you never even have to go to the gym to get the amount of exercise proved to improve your health, though a gym can often help. This chapter will give you the knowledge of why physical activity is beneficial and how you can get moving to enjoy those results.

Physical Activity Benefits Heart Health

People are designed to be active creatures. Not so long ago, people had to perform physical work to feed, clothe, and shelter themselves. Modern living has changed all of that, but it cannot change the fundamental need of people to move and use their bodies in order to maintain optimum functioning. As average levels of physical activity have declined, medical professionals have observed an accompanying decline in the body's physical functioning. Researchers are also studying the relationship of physical inactivity with a decline in mental functioning.

Numerous studies now substantiate the fact that a minimal amount of physical movement is not only beneficial but essential. Many aspects of aging, such as the loss of strength, balance, and the ability to move and care for oneself, were formerly viewed as a natural result of the aging process. Research today shows that many of these consequences are not actually the result of aging. Rather, they are the result of disuse of the body and a failure to take advantage of its physical capabilities. To retain your vitality and energy, you need to keep yourself physically active.

How Does Activity Affect the Heart?

Physical inactivity is a major risk factor for heart disease. The heart is a muscle that benefits from regular use to keep it and the circulatory system healthy. When a person is inactive, the heart muscle is weaker. With each beat, an unfit heart muscle pumps a lower volume of blood than a stronger, fit heart.

Because less blood is pumped, the heart has to beat more frequently to ensure adequate circulation of blood around the body. This more rapid heart rate can also result in an increase in blood pressure over time, causing stiffness and hardening of the arteries and affecting the health of the circulatory system. In contrast, when the heart is strong and healthy, stroke volume is strong. The heart rate is slower, and a more healthy tone is maintained in the arterial walls.

Increasing physical activity leads to an increase in the levels of HDL, or good cholesterol. This change is independent of any weight loss that may also occur as increased activity burns up more calories. Physical activity also lowers LDL and triglyceride levels.

Studies show that regular physical activity not only lowers bad cholesterol and triglycerides and increases good cholesterol, but that it also reduces risk of death from all causes, reduces feelings of depression and anxiety, and helps build and maintain healthy bones, muscles, and joints.

Only moderate amounts of physical activity are required to reverse the downward spiral toward ill health. A moderate amount of activity can mean as little as thirty minutes of brisk walking on most days of the week.

It's clear that physical activity provides countless benefits. If you are particularly concerned about the health of your heart and your cholesterol levels, regular activity is one of the best things you can do for yourself.

Studies also show that people who are physically active after a first heart attack have a significantly lower risk of having a second heart attack when compared with people who remained inactive.

How Much Activity Is Necessary?

According to guidelines issued by the U.S. Surgeon General, the U.S. Department of Health and Human Services, and the National Heart, Lung, and Blood Institute, the minimum amount of activity for health includes the following factors:

- Should continue for at least thirty minutes total
- Can be accumulated in bouts as short as eight to ten minutes
- Should be of moderate intensity, such as brisk walking
- Should occur on most, preferably all, days of the week
- Should include some resistance exercise and stretching during the week

The guidelines also note that more activity and a higher intensity will provide greater health and fitness benefits. The general guidelines listed above set forth minimum amounts of activity necessary to enjoy health benefits. Clearly, this level of exercise will not prepare you to run a marathon or to climb Mount Everest, but such events may not be among your immediate goals. You may simply want to feel better and know you are doing something good for your health. The message for you is loud and clear—with moderate amounts of physical activity on a regular basis, you can achieve this goal.

ALERT

According to surveys, only 40 percent of adults meet the minimum activity recommendation to provide health benefits of thirty minutes on most days of the week.

What Is Moderate Activity?

Research shows that activity can come in a variety of ways and still provide health benefits. The good news is that with so many activities to choose from, you are likely to find something that you enjoy and are able to incorporate into your life on a regular basis. The following are examples of moderate amounts of physical activity:

▼ **EXAMPLES OF MODERATE AMOUNTS OF ACTIVITIES**

Types of Activity	Length of Time
Playing volleyball	45 minutes
Playing touch football	30–45 minutes
Walking 1¾ miles	35 minutes (20-minute mile, or pace of 3 miles/hour)
Basketball (shooting baskets)	30 minutes
Bicycling 5 miles	30 minutes
Walking 2 miles	30 minutes (15-minute mile, or pace of 4 miles/hour)
Water aerobics	30 minutes
Swimming laps	20 minutes
Wheelchair basketball	20 minutes

You can also perform some activities that are performed at a higher intensity, such as bicycling, jumping rope, running, shoveling snow, or climbing stairs for a shorter amount of time (fifteen minutes or so) to get similar results. However, it is not necessary to do high-intensity exercises to achieve health benefits, particularly those associated with improvements in cholesterol levels. Moderate-intensity exercise can improve heart health. The most important thing is to get moving!

Once you initiate an exercise routine it becomes easier to maintain, but that does not necessarily mean you will not still need to exert some effort to keep things up. The key to maintaining an exercise regimen is to find something that you can and will do regularly and that you do it for at least thirty minutes on most days of the week. Remember that you can break up those thirty minutes. For example, you can take a ten-minute morning walk, run a quick errand on a bicycle at noon for ten minutes, and then take another ten-minute walk at the end of the day. That adds up to a total of thirty minutes in one day. Again, you are not capped at thirty minutes. The more you do, the better!

Lifestyle Activity Is Important

Many people are so conditioned into thinking that exercise means going to the gym that they forget that everyday life presents them with numerous opportunities to get active during the day. If you have time to go to the gym, that's fantastic. But if you don't, do not despair. You can create more movement opportunities during your day that make a difference. Look for every opportunity for activity. Make a schedule. Give up TV time. Do whatever it takes to find time for activity.

Here are some examples of lifestyle activity:

- Walk to run an errand in the neighborhood, rather than taking a car.
- Play outdoor games with children instead of watching television together.
- Park farther away from the shop.
- Get off the train or bus one stop early and walk the rest of the way.
- Carry your groceries to your car or load them into your car yourself.
- Wash your car instead of taking it to the car wash.
- Rake leaves instead of using a leaf blower.
- Get up to switch appliances on or off instead of always using the remote control.

- Ride a bicycle for transportation instead of driving a car.
- Do some vigorous housecleaning, such as vacuuming, sweeping, or mopping.

Be creative. Find more and more ways that you can move during your day. These activities all add up and make a difference. For example, according to estimates for a 150-pound person, standing up for three ten-minute phone calls will burn twenty calories. In contrast, sitting for thirty minutes during those three phone calls burns only four calories. Simply by standing for those brief intervals, you have created a sixteen-calorie deficit. While sixteen calories may not seem like much, when it is repeated hour after hour, day after day, it and other small actions start to mean the difference between unwanted pounds and maintaining your ideal weight. If you added walking or pacing to your phone calls, it would even provide greater benefits. You may recall that after you eat during the day, your blood is filled with sugars and fats, blood glucose and triglycerides. These are sources of fuel that you can use immediately. However, if you are not active and do not use up this energy, it ends up ultimately stored as fat. One of the keys to keeping all systems healthy is to use up this fuel for its intended purpose and stimulate your heart, lungs, muscles, and skeletal and nervous systems. So get active after those meals, though not too active right after, of course.

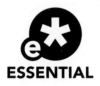

ESSENTIAL

If you can make time for regular workouts in a gym, that's great. Keep in mind, however, that studies show that people who live an otherwise sedentary life and work out for one hour per day are not burning as many calories as people who do not go to the gym but who take part in lifestyle activities throughout the day. Constantly look for more activity opportunities in life in general, whether more walking breaks, sports activities, or just activities around the home.

Exercise Your Way to a Healthy Heart

One of the best forms of exercise that provides a healthful challenge for the human body is walking. It is economical, easy to fit into your day, bears a low risk of injury, and is effective in improving health. Numerous studies show that people who walk regularly have less risk of death or disability from disease.

Studies have shown that people who participate in regular walking programs have higher levels of HDL cholesterol, lower levels of total and LDL cholesterol, and lower levels of triglycerides or blood fats. In addition to reducing these risks of heart disease, walking helps you to enjoy many other benefits, including maintaining a healthy weight, improving the condition of bones and muscles, and reducing stress and tension.

FACT

A study showed that older men who started walking about two miles a day had a 50 percent lower risk of heart attack than men who walked only a quarter mile. In addition, the study found that the risk of a heart attack dropped an additional 15 percent for every additional half mile walked per day.

Your Exercise Program: The First Steps

You're ready to get going with your daily exercise, but you're not quite sure how to begin. That's natural. A regular exercise program does include a few details that you need to address. The following information provides you with everything you need to know to get moving.

Check with Your Health Care Provider

Before you get started with any exercise program, it is a good idea to check with your health care provider. If you are apparently healthy and under the age of sixty-five, then a moderate exercise program is probably fine. If, however, you are older or have any known chronic conditions such as arthritis, diabetes, or heart disease, you need to check with your health care provider. An exercise program is likely to have multiple benefits for you, but safe is always better than sorry. Check with your doctor in case there are any specific limitations that require your awareness.

Find the Right Shoes

Your most important and significant investment is in the shoes that you will wear. Take the time to find a comfortable, sturdy shoe that fits the needs of your foot and provides good arch support. Shoe technology these days is actually quite sophisticated. Go to a reputable athletic footwear store that allows returns if the shoe is not a good fit for you.

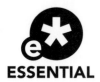

ESSENTIAL

If you plan to exercise both at home and at the office, consider investing in two pairs of shoes. This way you can always leave a pair at work. Otherwise, you will have to carry your shoes daily. It's important to make getting active as easy as possible. Again, while this represents a bigger investment in the beginning, it will pay multiple dividends over time in your improved health and quality of life.

Consider eventually buying shoe inserts. Today's shoes do not come with insoles that last as long as the outer part of the shoe. Yet, the cushioning that provides you with support is essential to keep you comfortable and to prevent injury. When you purchase your shoes, ask the salesperson to also help you to find an appropriate insole. This will make a tremendous difference in your long-term comfort.

Choose the Right Clothing and Accessories

As far as sportswear for exercise, you want to wear fabrics that breathe, such as cotton or polyester blends. Many modern fabrics also feature wicking qualities that draw your perspiration away from your skin. This can enhance your walking comfort. Women who need the extra support should wear an athletic sports bra. Comfort is your primary objective.

Sun protection is also important. Be sure to wear sunscreen. A hat is also a good idea to protect your face. Depending on how sensitive you are to sun exposure, you may want to purchase a hat that also shields the back of your neck. Sunglasses provide coverage for your eyes. Choose a pair that is lightweight and comfortable. More than anything, you want your walks as enjoyable as possible. Find the accessories that work best for you.

Stay Hydrated

Staying properly hydrated is essential for good health. If you are exercising for longer than an hour and are not near a water fountain, bringing your own water supply is a good idea. Some companies market fanny packs that serve as water bottle carriers that are handy for longer walks. Most important, remember to drink plenty of fluids before, during, and after your exercise. For moderate levels of exercise, plan on about five to seven ounces of water every fifteen to twenty minutes.

Consider a Pedometer

It is not necessary to purchase a pedometer, but it is a great tool to measure your progress and keep you motivated. You should take at least 10,000 steps a day, the equivalent of about five miles, but as always, more is better. The steps the pedometer measures do not require a particular intensity level or a specific duration. What they represent is that you have maintained a level of daily activity that contributes to your health.

The motivational aspect of the pedometer is that it helps you realize exactly how much you move around during the day. If you've had a busy, active day, you can supplement that with a short walk to reach your daily goal. If you've had a fairly inactive day, then you can save time for a longer walk. You can constantly try to increase the number of steps you take daily and break your old records. This can help you become a more active person on a daily basis, which can make a significant difference in your overall caloric expenditure as well as your health and well-being.

Your Walking Program

You can walk indoors at a shopping mall or on a treadmill. You can walk outdoors through your neighborhood, around the office, or at local parks or schools. You can walk alone or use the exercise as a time to catch up with friends or even to conduct business. You can use it to enhance your recreational pursuits, such as golfing or hiking, or you can simply do it as a way to stay in shape. You can walk any way you wish. To get the most out of your walking, consider trying the following to both feel great and avoid injury.

Walking Warm-Up

When you begin, start out at a comfortable pace. Let your arms hang naturally at your sides so they swing rhythmically with each step. Stand tall and maintain good posture. After about five minutes of walking, if you enjoy performing some stretches to make your walk more comfortable, you can. Research shows, however, that pre-exercise stretching does not prevent injury. At the same time, it does not do any harm, so if you find it comfortable, go ahead and incorporate a few stretches. Do not hold the stretches for more than ten to twenty seconds, however, as you do not want to cool down and lose the benefits of your warm-up. After you complete your stretches, you can continue with your walk.

Walking Technique

Posture is the most important aspect of walking technique. Stand tall with your ears above your shoulders, arms at your sides, shoulders above hips, and abdominal muscles slightly pulled in to actively support your lower back. If you want to increase the intensity of your walk, bend your elbows and swing your arms more vigorously. Take more steps, rather than longer strides. Keep your focus ahead to maintain good posture. Let your heel strike first and push forward through the ball of your foot. Keep your elbows in and avoid swinging your arms across your body.

Walking Cooldown

After you finish the more brisk portion of your walk, take time to slowly bring your body back to the way it felt when you began. Gradually slow back down to the comfortable pace you started out with. By the time you stop walking, you should have relaxed breathing and a calm heart rate. You need to spend only a few minutes on your walking cooldown, but it's important to take this time.

After your walk is a great time to include some final stretches. Unlike the beginning of your walk, your muscles are warm and ready to enjoy a long stretch. Good stretches to perform include shoulder rolls for the neck and shoulders, a standing calf stretch for the back of the lower leg, hamstring stretch for the back of the upper leg, standing side stretch for the side of the torso, and standing cat stretch to release the lower back. Breathe deeply, and hold each stretch anywhere from twenty to thirty seconds. Enjoy your stretches and your feeling of accomplishment. You have just improved your health. You deserve to enjoy it and feel good about yourself.

Step It Up

Walking is a great form of exercise suitable for nearly anyone, anytime, and anywhere. It's not the only form of exercise that is beneficial, though. Changing places and routes can help keep walking interesting, but to stay engaged you may need other exercises to do. Once you feel comfortable walking you may wish to take your exercise routine to the next level. Remember, while getting any exercise is good, more is better. Working at a greater intensity, for a longer duration, or doing a combination of exercises will all help to boost your routine.

Why Walk When You Can Run?

Have you ever looked at someone running and admired them or thought, "I wish I could do that." Most people, in fact, can. Of course, certain people have true physical disabilities that prevent them from taking a jog, such as severe arthritis or heart and lung conditions. For the rest, taking that first run is not impossible, just hard. That first run may be only fifty yards. Every day, though, that run can get a little longer, a little faster, until you are the person others are admiring. Remember, no one was born with the ability to run for miles. That means that all the runners you see made the decision to continue their efforts. They may not have enjoyed it the first, second, or thirtieth time, but nearly everyone who runs repeatedly enjoys it at some point.

Running follows many of the same rules for other exercise, with increased importance of the shoes and clothes, the latter preferably light, and if running in the dark, reflective. Running is one of the best forms of exercise, as it allows for sustained periods of movement. It helps expand your lungs, strengthens your heart and your leg muscles, and burns massive amounts of calories. In addition to its effectiveness, running is one of the most flexible and easiest exercises to take up. All you need is a pair of shoes, some comfortable clothing, and somewhere safe to run. You can do it anytime and nearly anywhere. All you need to do is put one foot in front of the other and see where your feet take you.

Why Run When You Can Fly?

Once you get lighter on your feet, you will feel comfortable doing all sorts of things you never thought you could do. You may start walking at a brisker pace naturally. You may suddenly want to play sports, run with your children, or even run a 5K. Remember, movement breeds movement. It's up to you to get things started and keep things going, but your body will do its share by rewarding you with limitless opportunities. The more you do, the higher your HDL, the lower your LDL, and the lower your triglycerides. Exercise also reduces blood pressure, blood sugar, and stress, further improving your health.

Overall, the more intense and active you are, the better you will feel. This improved feeling will not just affect your body, looks, and health, but also your overall mood. Exercise releases natural endorphins and neurotransmitters that carry with you to all aspects of your life, without the side effects and addiction to pharmacology. Your better health and mood will influence all aspects of your life, from your career to your family. Obviously, do not start exercising with the intention of soon completing an "iron man" triathlon, but there is value in exploring the next level of activity. Perhaps you are the type of person who gets bored during long walks or runs. Fortunately, there are plenty of other options.

Sports

Not everyone enjoys long periods of doing the same activity like walking or running, but nearly everyone enjoys games. Sports combine the enjoyment of games with the benefits of exercise. Moreover, there are hundreds of active sports to choose from. Here are some common favorites, as well as some you may not have considered:

- Baseball/Softball
- Basketball
- Football/Rugby
- Hockey/Field Hockey

- Tennis/Racquetball/Badminton
- Soccer
- Ultimate Frisbee
- Golf/Frisbee Golf

There are hundreds more, but these are some of the most common competitive sports out there. Because of their ubiquity, it is much easier to find leagues, clubs, and facilities that support these sports. The important thing is to find what you like. If you enjoy what you are playing, you will not think about the length and intensity of your exercise, which will lead to a longer, more intense workout. This increase in exercise will further support all aspects of your health. Remember, it's not whether you win or lose, it's that you got healthier and had fun doing it!

Weight Lifting

Sustaining a brisk pace and steady heart rate is not the only important form of exercise. Increasing your strength is important, too. By increasing your muscle mass, not only do you convert the calories of protein into muscle, but also your new muscle needs calories to function, increasing your metabolism. Lifting weights is one of the most efficient forms of building muscle.

ALERT

More and more research suggests lifting weights may be one of the most efficient forms of losing weight. Not only are calories required to perform the exercise, but calories are also needed to build muscle. In addition, muscle has a higher metabolism than fat, so people with more muscle have a higher metabolism and burn more calories, even at rest.

For many, weight lifting, like running, can seem intimidating. They picture muscular bodybuilders lifting massive amounts of weight while groaning and looking at their smaller selves in disgust. This cannot be further from the truth. While there are still some gyms that cater to the intense bodybuilder, most now cater to the general population. Most gyms, like the

YMCA and many commercial health clubs, serve the regular person who just wants to be healthier and get in shape. Health clubs are filled with young and old, large and skinny, longtime lifters and those brand-new to the practice. Most gyms are very nonjudgmental places.

Once you get over your fears and join a gym, the challenge is learning what to do. Many may find free weights, or weights not attached to a machine, intimidating at first, so the best way to start is on gym machines. Most gym machines show the exercise you can do right on them, so you can simply follow the instructions. If you still feel uncomfortable, you can do your first or several workouts with a personal trainer who can show you some basic exercises. Once you get comfortable on machines, you can try "hybrid" machines, or machines where the resistance used is free weights. While you are getting comfortable on these machines, pay attention to those around you. Other people can serve as great instructors, as you can simply watch them.

Eventually, you may feel comfortable using totally free weights, including barbells and dumbbells. The benefit of these weights is that since they are free, you must use stabilizing "accessory" muscles that you may not need to use with machines. Start with light weights and work your way up. Remember, when lifting heavier weights, use a spotter, a person who can grab the weight if you feel unable to lift it, for safety reasons. The last thing you want is for a dropped weight to scare you away from this invaluable activity.

You do not have to go to a health club to work out with weights. Sports stores sell weights you can buy. These are relatively expensive compared with gym memberships and can occupy a lot of space in the home. If exercising at home is the only way you will work out, then the cost is more than worth it in terms of the dividends for your health.

Cross-Training

Many of the benefits of exercise come from the body having to undergo a new experience. When you start walking, running, weight lifting, or doing any other sport, your body gets exposed to new movements and strains. The human body has learned to accommodate to new stresses by adjusting itself to respond to that stress. When you lift weights, your body responds

to the stress on your muscles by building more muscle. When you perform cardiovascular exercise, your body responds by the heart building
more muscle to accommodate to the need for increased blood flow. Other
changes occur as well. In addition to your muscles and heart, other areas of
your body also strengthen. Your bones, tendons, and ligaments all restruc-
ture to increase their strength. You build more oxygen-carrying red blood
cells and oxygen-transporting blood vessels. The body's response to the
work of exercise is to make it stronger, and this new strength benefits all
aspects of your life.

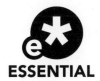

ESSENTIAL

Cross-training not only gives the sustained excitement of different exercises to your mind and body, but also allows you to reap the benefits of every form of exercise. You can strengthen your heart, open
your lungs, and build the different muscle types used for quick movements and sustained activity.

To get the most benefit, you should allow your body exposure to different stresses. While any amount of moderate exercise is very beneficial, the
most benefit comes from doing different forms of exercises. Serious weight
lifters and runners follow this strategy. Weight lifters are always changing
their movements and therefore how they stress their muscles. This produces the greatest muscle growth from the constant accommodation to
new strains. Runners will vary paces and distances to maximize stress on
different types of muscle fibers.

Of course, if you are starting from a position of no exercise, then you
should start with one new activity. As you get comfortable in that activity
and pursue it to a level where you feel you are reaping a significant benefit,
then you may realize even greater benefit by seeking out new forms of exercise. Not only will this maximize the benefit to your body, but it will also
help stave off boredom and encourage motivation.

The benefits of exercise cannot be overstated. Exercise improves your
entire cholesterol profile, including raising your HDL, lowering your LDL,
and lowering your triglycerides. Exercise also reduces your blood pressure,
lowers your blood sugar, makes you slimmer, and decreases stress. All of

these independently reduce your risk for cardiovascular disease. Therefore, by exercising, you make a tremendous reduction in the likelihood of suffering a heart attack or stroke. You should have a goal of at least thirty minutes total of moderate exercise at least three times per week. By getting active, you will boost your health, look better, have more energy, and improve your mood. The benefits are innumerable to you and those around you. So get out there, and get moving!

CHAPTER 11

Stress Management for a Healthy Heart

Stress. Even the sound of the word evokes feelings of tension. Stress is a daily aspect of modern living. Stress can keep you motivated and even save your life. If unmanaged, however, stress can kill you. Excess stress weakens the immune system. Furthermore, stress can make any disease condition worse. In this chapter, you will discover what stress is, how stress contributes to heart disease, how you can identify stress, and what steps you can take to reduce stress and restore balance to your life.

What Is Stress?

Stress is actually a natural physiological response to something that triggers a feeling of fear or threat. This response, called "fight or flight," is designed to help you to survive life-threatening situations. The natural chemical response that affects your mind and body is like a miracle drug that can help save your life in the face of a dangerous emergency. For example, if your house catches on fire in the middle of the night, stress can help you to think fast and effectively the minute you wake up. As soon as you realize you are in danger, stress gives you energy to jump out of bed and run for your life. You have extra strength to save loved ones who are possibly in danger. In an instant, your mind is alert, your heart is pounding, your muscles are strong, and you have superhuman energy.

The Stress Response

The body's response to stress is stimulated by stress hormones, like adrenaline and cortisol, released by your body to prepare you for action. Among other things, these stress hormones do the following:

- Increase your heart rate and blood pressure to pump an extra burst of oxygen-rich blood around your body so you can get moving
- Stop the flow of blood to your digestive system and skin by constricting arteries, saving blood flow for more needed areas
- Channel the increased blood flow to the brain and muscles by relaxing arteries
- Increase perspiration to cool the body
- Activate receptors that generate quick bursts of energy
- Speed up your breathing rate and open bronchial tubes to draw more oxygen-rich air into the lungs

When you look at all of these changes, it's easy to see how this chemically induced state of emergency preparedness is extremely useful in life-threatening situations.

The modern challenge, however, is to manage the stress response, which can trigger when you're not in any physical danger at all. In fact, most contemporary stresses are mental and emotional. You find yourself stuck in traffic, missing deadlines at work, getting ready to make a presentation, or worrying that your child won't make the soccer team. You worry about your family, your money, and for those reading this book, your health. For some people, these stress levels stay high throughout the day. Both body and mind feel the strain, and the body gets no opportunity to physically release any of this tension energy.

ESSENTIAL

The stress response protects the body in a number of ways. It triggers the body to release blood sugar into the bloodstream to provide immediately available energy for fuel. It beefs up the blood-clotting mechanism in the event of any potential injury. In addition, your body becomes extremely alert to enable you to spot immediately any signs of danger.

How Stress Harms Health

Stress can harm health if it mounts to levels at which you feel that you can no longer cope. This usually occurs after stress levels have remained high over a prolonged period of time.

The hormones released during stressful situations, like adrenaline and cortisol, raise blood sugar and constrict many of your blood vessels. This raises your blood pressure, increasing your cardiovascular risk. The increased blood sugar and hormones increase your LDL cholesterol and triglycerides while decreasing your HDL. In other words, like smoking, obesity, or lack of exercise, stress affects all aspects of your cholesterol profile and increases your cardiovascular risk.

Other physical and mental symptoms of excessive stress include rapid pulse, chronic muscle tension, headaches, digestive problems, ulcers, infections, irritability, depression, anxiety, loss of ability to concentrate, altered sleeping or eating habits, and increased use of drugs or alcohol. Understanding stress and having skills to manage stress effectively, therefore, are important to your overall health and wellness.

Stress and Heart Disease

The American Heart Association does not include stress as one of the leading risk factors for heart disease. However, this may have more to do with the difficulty of separating stress from other risk factors, since stress contributes to various risk factors. In other words, it is difficult to prove that stress is an independent risk factor given that it also contributes to so many other risk factors, including smoking, physical inactivity, overeating, and high cholesterol, blood sugar, and blood pressure. The American Heart Association, however, does note that individual responses to stress may be a contributing factor to heart disease risk.

Stress and Heart Function

After studying the long-term effects of stress, some researchers believe that prolonged stress can cause damage to blood vessels. Stress hormones, to channel blood flow to essential areas in times of stress, will constrict these vessels. This constriction leads to endothelial dysfunction, a precursor to the development of atherosclerosis.

Over time, the blood vessels lose their ability to dilate effectively until they cannot respond appropriately to changes in blood demands. For example, constricted arteries would fail to provide an increased blood flow to meet the needs of working muscles in the legs or to meet the increased demands of blood flow to a heart that is pumping more vigorously to support physical activity.

Identifying Stress in Your Life

Most contemporary stress-inducing situations are not dangerous in and of themselves. What makes them stressful is the way you react to them. Some people thrive in situations that make others miserably tense and anxious. For example, you may hate meeting deadlines, while a friend works productively under that type of pressure. If you are frequently rushed or competitive and feel overwhelmed by this, or you let small frustrations get to you, or you find it hard to forget your worries and relax, tackling your stress levels will most likely improve your health. At the same time, you can certainly make your life more enjoyable.

Other types of stress are not caused by your attitude but are rather the product of a busy life. For example, if you are driving in heavy traffic and someone quickly cuts in front of you, that is a stressful situation. You have a legitimate fear for your safety, as a car accident could result. Your reaction, however, does not require you to burn off any physical energy. Rather, you remain seated in your car. You are likely to tighten your muscles and experience feelings of tension and anxiety as your body undergoes the physiological and biochemical changes associated with the "fight or flight" response.

ALERT

Numerous studies demonstrate that people who are more likely to become angry have about three times greater risk of having a heart attack or sudden cardiac death than those who are less prone to become angry. Other studies show that as people experience anger, they are more likely to have an arrhythmia, or irregular heartbeat.

Often, when you feel "stressed out," it is a generalized feeling of stress. If you take a moment to examine your situation, however, you will find that your feelings are actually the cumulative result of numerous individual pressures that have finally reached the boiling point. One of the first steps toward learning how to manage stress effectively is to identify these individual pressures—the types of things in your life that cause you stress. Your awareness is the first step.

The next time you start to feel overwhelmed and stressed out, explore these feelings in greater depth. Ask yourself the following questions to determine what is causing these emotions:

- Am I overcommitted?
- Am I taking care of others and neglecting my own self-care?
- Am I trying to accomplish everything on my own without asking for any support from anyone else?
- Are my expectations unrealistic?
- What is going on in my life right now that gives me a sense of struggle?
- Is what I stress over more important than my health and happiness?

If you are the type of person who finds it helpful to keep a journal, try to record things that trigger your stress. Write down what happened, what you were thinking or feeling, and how you reacted physically. This can give you valuable insight into the cumulative triggers you face throughout the day. Then consider the importance of those things and the importance of your long-term health and well-being. Consider the effects of stress on your health and mood and how that then affects those around you. Is what you stress over more concerning than premature death and disability? If not, then it is worth learning how to manage your stress.

ESSENTIAL

When you start to identify the causes for your feelings and you also note how you react to these stressors, you bring more awareness and understanding to your personal situation. Once you realize what triggers your stress, then you are ready to consider taking realistic steps to cope with your personal matters.

Strategies for Dealing with Stress

It's important for your health and mental wellness that you feel a sense of control over your life. Stress management and relaxation are learned skills, and they require strategies for success. The strategies discussed in this section can help you manage stress successfully.

It's important to make time to learn stress management skills and relaxation techniques. Learning how to manage stress or how to eliminate some of the stressors in your life is important when it comes to keeping your immune system strong, reducing your risk of illness, and improving your feelings of well-being.

Identify Priorities and Manage Time Effectively

Time management is a critical skill to develop to successfully manage stress. Everyone has the same number of hours in the day. Some people, however, are more effective managers of their time and priorities. To get organized, first identify your priorities. Next, make a realistic plan for how long it will take to get things done. Do the best that you can, and remember to also leave time for yourself.

If you feel that you need help in this area, consider taking a course in time or stress management. Consult your health care provider about available resources. You may want to enroll in a group course or work one-on-one with a counselor.

Rely on Social Support

Social support is a very important factor in effective stress management. Friends and family can help you to talk over troublesome topics and help you keep your perspective. Take time to make friends and to maintain relationships. Even a cherished pet can provide you with companionship and dispel feelings of loneliness and isolation.

If you feel you need more support, go ahead and ask for help from others in your home, workplace, or community. Your employer may have an employee assistance program that can provide you with confidential counseling. Your church or community center may also have helpful resources. Make it a priority to develop relationships with people who influence your life positively.

Numerous studies have shown the positive effect of relationships on stress and health. Prioritizing and fostering those relationships is important not only for those around you, but for yourself as well. The more close ties you have with your family, friends, and community, the greater benefit to your health and happiness. Studies even indicate that pet ownership can contribute to heart health. Researchers have found that pet owners consistently have reduced stress reactions as measured by lower heart rates and blood pressures, especially when the pets are present.

Forgiveness is important to coping with difficult emotions. Negative feelings and stressful situations can adversely affect your health. When you forgive others for actions that you feel were unfair or inappropriate, you can release or heal strong negative emotions. It's important to learn coping skills that include how to let go of negative feelings and restore your peace of mind. Also remember how you appreciate receiving forgiveness. Share that feeling of receiving forgiveness with others.

Express Yourself Without Anger

Remember that people who get angry easily are much more likely to die from a heart attack. If you find that you are often irritated or annoyed, learn constructive methods to deal with disagreeable situations. Learn more effective communication skills to defuse conflicts. Make sure that you are not allowing resentment to build up inside you. Over time, denial of anger can lead to unhealthy blow-ups or chronic negative feelings. The healthiest approach is to learn how to effectively express your feelings in positive and constructive ways.

It may help to remember some simple alternatives to becoming angry or frustrated in stressful situations. If possible, leave the scene of a stressful situation before it gets to you. Talk to someone you trust about how you feel, or take some time on your own to brainstorm nonstressful ways to respond to a stressful issue. Most important, remember to breathe deeply and ask yourself, "In the scheme of things, does this really matter? Is this more important than my health and happiness?"

Nature Outings

Studies show that spending time in nature promotes feelings of calm and relaxation. When you look at a beautiful sunset, enjoy the sounds of the pounding surf, or enjoy a beautiful view from the side of a mountain, the vastness of the world helps to put all the small frustrations back in the proper perspective. Find something active outside that you enjoy, and take time to put it in your schedule. You can incorporate nature with physical activity such as running, walking, or other activities and sports. Remember, regular physical activity is an important health behavior that can return multiple dividends. Not only will you feel better, look great, and manage your weight effectively, but you also will manage stress better by being active on a regular basis. Something as simple as a short walk can provide a powerful positive outlet for tension.

Make Time for Self-Care

One of the biggest contributors to feelings of stress is the sense that life is out of control. To avoid this, make time for yourself, just like taking time to exercise or eat healthy. You deserve time for your own self-care. For one thing, it supports your health, which in turn helps you to better support those you care about. Take a moment to identify things that you enjoy, that bring you pleasure, and that are fun and restorative. Make it a point to incorporate these activities into your schedule.

It is never easy to change a habit. Unless stress is managed and the reasons for maintaining the behavioral change are foremost in your mind, old habits prevail. A calm, clear, and focused mind and a healthy, realistic attitude are important for achieving any goal. This holds equally true for the incorporation of healthy lifestyle habits.

Restoring Health Through Relaxation

Research suggests that relaxation techniques can be used to counteract the stress response, with significant health benefits. Regular relaxation can reduce blood cortisol levels, blood pressure, cholesterol, and blood glucose.

Clinical trials show that relaxation can reduce headaches, pain, anxiety, and menopausal symptoms. At the same time, it can enhance healing, immune cell response, concentration, and feelings of well-being. It has even been shown to improve fertility rates in infertile women.

Research done in the 1970s by Dr. Herbert Benson of Harvard University began to explore the relationship between mental techniques and physiological effects. Benson studied people who participated in transcendental meditation. He coined the term "the relaxation response," which is defined as "a calm state brought about by sitting quietly and repeating a sound, words, or muscular activity over and over. When everyday thoughts intrude, the person passively disregards them and returns to the repetition." The relaxation response reflects a physiological state brought about by reducing stress and calming the mind.

The following effects are the result of the relaxation response:

- Reduced blood pressure
- Reduced heart rate
- Slower breathing rate
- Restoration of blood flow to the extremities
- Reduction in perspiration
- Release of muscular tension

When you look at the results of the relaxation response and compare them with the list at the beginning of the chapter, it's easy to see how relaxation counteracts the stress response and restores the body to a state of balance.

As a result of numerous studies in this area, relaxation techniques are used to help people with problems such as hypertension and cardiac arrhythmias, among others. While these skills are useful for people who are managing chronic disease, they are also valuable for promoting health and preventing stress-related illnesses. Make time to explore and learn techniques that help you to relax. Some people use prayer, while others engage in practices like yoga or tai chi. Find the methods that work for you.

Relaxation and Deep Breathing

One of the easiest ways to achieve relaxation is to engage in deep, mindful breathing exercises. This can help to trigger the relaxation response. This type of exercise is easy to learn, fast to perform, and requires no equipment. As you continue to explore other methods of relaxation, use the following breathing exercise to help you ease tensions and restore your sense of balance and calm. It will do the health of your body, mind, and spirit a world of good. As you emerge from your restorative relaxation time, remind yourself that you have the power to create your own health and to enjoy all that life has to offer.

A Simple Breathing Exercise

This exercise is an excellent introduction to relaxation and to meditation techniques. It increases self- and body awareness. A two- to three-minute "breathing break" during the day is very restorative. To perform this simple exercise, sit or lie comfortably with your hands resting in your lap. Relax your muscles and close your eyes.

Make no effort to control your breath, simply breathe naturally. As you breathe in and out, focus your attention on the breath and how the body moves with each inhalation and exhalation.

Take a few moments to focus inward. Notice the movement of your body as you breathe. Observe your inhalation and exhalation. Pay particular attention to how the breath moves your body. Observe your chest, shoulders, rib cage, and belly. Notice subtleties such as whether the chest or belly rises with inhalation and how your body responds to exhalation. Don't try to control your breath, simply focus your attention on it. This singular focus brings you into the present moment and into the immediate experience of your body. It often results in slower, deeper breaths that further relax your body. Continue for two to three minutes and then gently open your eyes. Over time, you can lengthen the period of relaxation, if you prefer.

Restoring Life Through Meditation

For centuries, many have used meditation to reduce stress in their lives. The act of meditation is similar to relaxation in the attempt to let go of stressful thoughts. The key difference between meditation and relaxation is that during relaxation, one tries to passively empty the mind, while meditation represents active focus on certain thoughts through abandoning other thoughts.

Numerous studies have shown that meditation, like relaxation, improves health and mood. Meditation is also known to improve cognition and focus. Meditation produces many of the same physiologic changes as the relaxation response. Because of meditation's differences in practice of intense focus rather than lack of focus, meditation can better serve those who have difficulty emptying their mind and decompressing. Meditation can also be complementary. Similar to how varied exercises can further help your body, the most stress reduction is likely obtained by incorporating various practices that reduce stress. Not only do you obtain the benefits of each practice, but as with using different physical exercises to continue to develop and motivate the body, using different mental practices can help you continue to develop and motivate the mind.

Practicing Meditation

The practice of meditation can seem complex, but the basic concept is quite simple. The key, like relaxation, exercise, eating healthier, or changing or creating any other habit, is that it takes practice.

To begin, though you can commence nearly any time at any place, the ideal setting is to be in a quiet area, sitting comfortably. Sitting on the floor with your back straight tends to focus your attention further and is recommended but not necessary. Start to breathe in and out. Once in a rhythm, begin to focus your thoughts on an area that you would like to focus. Make that as specific an area as possible. You can focus on a certain aspect of your life, your family, your work, your health, or just simply focus on your breathing, being in the present moment. You may choose to concentrate on something that you like in your life and wish to augment, or you may choose to focus on that which you do not like and wish to correct.

What then makes meditation challenging is the other thoughts that enter your head. You may start to drift or hear a lot of background noise in your own mind. Recognize those other thoughts, do not get frustrated, and let go of those thoughts, bringing yourself back to where you originally wished to focus. This might seem simple, but you are constantly barraged with thoughts and stimuli throughout the day. Going even sixty seconds without allowing some new thought or stimulus is surprisingly challenging. With practice, you will notice you are able to focus for longer and longer periods. As with exercise, the more you do, the better it is for your health.

The highest yield of meditation is when you start your day and shortly before going to bed. Set a goal to practice for at least five minutes. You might set an alarm so you do not have to allow the intrusive thought of how long your meditation has lasted. You can derive significant benefit from five minutes, but once you are able to meditate that long without significant thought interruption, you may choose to practice even longer.

The Overall Benefits to You

With relaxation and meditation, many people feel they cannot spare the five minutes to obtain the significant benefit. Those who practice relaxation and meditation, though, know that the several minutes they spend incorporating either practice into their daily routine adds much more time to their lives. You will find it easier to focus, making you more productive. You will sleep better, making you feel more rested and able to do more. You will improve your cholesterol, blood pressure, and blood sugar, as well as feel more able to tackle other aspects of your health. This will add years to your life and improve the quality of those years. Those around you will appreciate your improved mood. Now you know that you can reduce stress nearly anytime, anywhere. Take the time now to get started!

CHAPTER 12

Smoke-Free for Heart Health

Smoking cigarettes greatly increases your risk of having a heart attack or stroke. Chemicals such as nicotine in cigarettes damage the lining of blood vessels and reduce HDL, or good cholesterol. In spite of the fact that nicotine is highly addictive, you can apply any of several strategies to successfully kick your smoking habit. The good news is that within minutes of your last cigarette, your body starts to change for the better.

The Harmful Effects of Smoking

You've probably already heard that smoking is bad for you. But do you really know what it can do? Consider the following facts. Smokers have a tremendously higher risk of lung diseases such as cancer, emphysema, bronchitis, and pulmonary fibrosis. Ever see people who have to walk around with an oxygen tank purely so they can breathe? Nearly all of those people became that way due to smoking. Imagine becoming out of breath after going only a few steps. Performing other tasks that help your life, like exercise, becomes tremendously harder.

Smoking also gives you a higher risk of nearly every form of cancer. In a healthy body, many areas have cells that go through a cycle of reproduction, where older cells die and newer cells take over. In cancer, some of the new cells have a genetic error where they end up replicating too much or living too long. The body makes more and more cells, ultimately creating a mass that can spread to invade your brain, lungs, liver, and bones. This is why people fear cancer, because for many, it can truly be a torturous way to live, and it can cause painful deaths.

FACT

Smoking is the cause of more than 440,000 deaths per year, according to the American Heart Association. This number represents more than one out of every six deaths!

Smoking also creates bad breath, impairs your sense of taste and smell, inflames gums, yellows teeth, and causes facial wrinkling and a more aged appearance. Smoking low-tar, low-nicotine, or menthol cigarettes does not reduce the risk of heart disease or negate any of the above consequences.

It Does Not Just Hurt You

Additional negative consequences of cigarette smoking for women include that it increases birth defects and reduces birth weight in infants born to smoking mothers, reduces fertility in women trying to get pregnant, and raises the risk of having a miscarriage or stillborn baby. Men who smoke have a higher incidence of erectile dysfunction. Exposure to cigarette smoke heightens the likelihood of children catching colds, infections, asthma, and respiratory ailments such as bronchitis and pneumonia, as well as children's long-term risk of pulmonary disease and cancer that affects many adults.

Studies confirm that secondhand smoke, or smoke absorbed by those not actually smoking, is also injurious. For the nonsmoker, secondhand smoke poses the same risks as inhaled smoke poses to the smoker because the lethal chemicals are in the smoke itself. Therefore, passive smoking or simply breathing smoke-filled air draws those same chemicals into the lungs and bloodstream. Secondhand smoke can often cause more harm, due to the lack of any sort of filtering in smoke from the back end of a cigarette.

Effects of Smoking on the Heart

When compared with nonsmokers, smokers have twice the risk of having a heart attack or stroke, and even higher risk when other risk factors are present. Furthermore, smokers who have a heart attack are much more likely to die. Smoking increases the risk of sudden cardiac death.

Cigarette smoking specifically harms the heart and circulatory system in a number of ways, including the following:

- Damaging the lining of the arteries
- Decreasing HDL cholesterol
- Accelerating plaque formation by increasing oxidation of LDL cholesterol
- Escalating heart rate and blood pressure by narrowing of the arteries
- Reducing the amount of available oxygen in the bloodstream by increasing levels of carbon monoxide, which compete with oxygen (and win) to bind with blood cells
- Raising the likelihood of blood clot formation

Blood vessels get stiffer when exposed to the toxins in cigarette smoke. Because of their stiffness, blood pressure increases. Also, blood vessels cannot dilate when necessary to meet increased oxygen and nutrient demands of organs, limiting blood flow to essential areas. This is a precursor to atherosclerosis, when progressive plaque causes blood vessel thinning.

Smoking cigarettes is not only harmful to your lungs, it is also very damaging to the health of your heart and circulatory system. In fact, more smokers die from heart attacks and strokes than from lung cancer or respiratory disease.

Nonsmokers exposed to environmental tobacco smoke are at a 25 percent higher relative risk of developing heart disease than nonsmokers not exposed to environmental tobacco smoke. According to the American Heart Association, approximately 40,000 nonsmokers die each year from cardiovascular disease resulting from exposure to passive tobacco smoke. While you may find it impossible to completely prevent exposure to secondhand smoke, you will benefit from avoiding it as much as you can.

The Benefits of Quitting

By quitting smoking, you reduce your risk of heart disease. At the same time, your odds of developing disease will continue to improve over the years. The benefits of quitting include less risk for numerous diseases, improved cholesterol and other lipid levels, and increased self-esteem and feelings of well-being. Quitting also benefits those around you who may suffer from consequences of secondhand smoke. Even if you believe that smoking in isolation cannot harm others, you track in many of the toxins on your body and clothing, which can still spread. If you smoke outside, you are spreading those toxins into the air that everyone breathes. If quitting for yourself is not enough, do it for others.

Quitting Improves Your Health

The health benefits of kicking the smoking habit truly start right away. Within twenty minutes of your last cigarette, nicotine is no longer causing constriction of blood vessels. As a result, your blood pressure decreases, your heart rate slows, and the temperature of your hands and feet rises as circulation improves. Within eight hours of your last cigarette, carbon monoxide levels drop in the bloodstream, and oxygen levels increase. Within twenty-four hours, the chances of having a heart attack are reduced. Within forty-eight hours, nerve endings begin to regenerate, and your sense of smell and taste start to return.

ALERT

Quitting the cigarette habit can improve your sex life. According to evidence from research, men who smoke fewer than ten cigarettes a day had a 16 percent higher risk of erectile dysfunction in comparison with men who had never smoked. Men who smoked more than one pack of cigarettes daily had a whopping 60 percent higher risk of erectile dysfunction when compared with nonsmokers.

During the first year of not smoking, your body continues to heal itself from the stress of absorbing the cigarette toxins. Coughing, sinus congestion, fatigue, and shortness of breath start to fade as the strength of the lungs is restored. After a smoke-free year, the increased risk from smoking is cut in half. With each passing year, the risk continues to diminish.

Quitting Saves Time and Money

Another great benefit of quitting is that you will save quite a bit of money by giving up the cigarette habit. Your savings come mostly from the fact that you no longer need to buy cigarettes. Since smoking increases your risk for so many diseases, you also save money by staying healthy and not creating huge medical bills. In addition, you no longer need to spend time and effort looking for or buying cigarettes, lighters, and matches, or searching for places to light up.

It Does Not Just Help You

Not only will your improved health and energy help yourself, it will help those around you. Loved ones who smoke may become more inclined to quit, and by quitting you decrease the chance that nonsmokers will pick up the habit. By decreasing secondhand smoke exposure to those around you, you will improve their health as well. Their risk of cardiovascular disease and cancer will lower significantly. Sometimes it's challenging to do things for yourself, but when you quit smoking, you are also doing something great for others.

Getting Ready to Give Up Cigarettes

Approximately 70 percent of adult smokers want to quit. Quitting, however, is not easy. Many smokers try multiple times before they eventually succeed. Thorough preparation can increase your odds of achieving a smoke-free future. The federal government provides resources to assist people. In a program set forth on the website *www.smokefree.gov*, the preparatory phase consists of five steps represented by the acronym "START."

The five steps are the following:

S = Set a quit date.
T = Tell family, friends, and coworkers that you plan to quit.
A = Anticipate and plan for the challenges that you will face.
R = Remove cigarettes and other tobacco products from your home, car, and work.
T = Talk to your doctor about getting help to quit.

The following sections examine each of these steps in detail.

Set a Quit Date

Once you have your mind made up that the benefits of not smoking far outweigh the risks of smoking, then you are ready to set a quit date. Know that you are genuinely ready to make this commitment before you decide upon your quit date. Choose a specific day at least two weeks in advance. This gives you plenty of time to prepare, without losing your motivation to quit. Choose a day when you're best positioned to take that essential first step, such as when you are with others who can support you or at a place where you cannot get easy access to cigarettes.

If you smoke at work, it may make things easier on you if you select either a weekend or vacation day to get started. Or, to make the occasion more memorable, select a special occasion such as your birthday, anniversary, or a national holiday.

Tell Others Your Plan

Social support is the single most important factor in determining whether you are successful in changing poor habits into good ones. The help of your family and friends makes changing any behavioral pattern much easier. Share your quitting plans with those who are close to you to solicit their support. It's often much harder to let others down than it is to let yourself down. Use peer pressure to your advantage.

The National Cancer Institute offers a smoking cessation guide with several helpful tips for developing your support system. First of all, the institute advises you to remind friends that your moods may change. Let them know that the longer you go without cigarettes, the sooner you will return to your old self. Also, if you have a friend or family member close to you who also smokes, see if he or she is interested in quitting with you. If not, ask him or her not to smoke around you. Seek out an ex-smoker to give you encouragement and advice during your tough moments.

Anticipate Challenges and Plan Ahead

Most people tend to form habitual patterns of smoking, such as immediately after a meal or when enjoying an alcoholic drink. These are the times that will present you with the strongest cravings. In addition to emotional cravings, most smokers also experience withdrawal symptoms including mood swings, feelings of irritability and depression, anxiety or restlessness, insomnia, headaches, difficulty concentrating, and increased hunger.

These symptoms are worst the first few weeks, and they are extremely powerful during the first week of quitting. To help manage the cravings, use the time before you quit to concentrate on the moments you observe that you want a cigarette most. Note when you have a cigarette and how you are feeling at the time. Then consider alternative ways to cope with those feelings and alternative activities during those times. For example, instead of having a cigarette after a meal, chew gum, drink water, squirt your mouth with breath spray, or brush your teeth. Be proactive in planning these alternatives, and buy the gum, breath spray, or whatever else you will need before you get to your scheduled quitting day.

FACT

Consider joining a support group, either in person, on the phone, or in an Internet chat room. You can check with the American Cancer Society, the Heart Association, or Lung Association for leads on groups that you can join. Social support can provide a great way to help you quit.

If it is helpful to you to keep a journal, write down your observations. An even easier way to create this record of your smoking pattern is to wrap a piece of paper around your pack of cigarettes and secure it with a rubber band. Every time that you have a cigarette, write down the time of day, place, and your reason for having the cigarette. Later, take the list that you have created and write down alternative strategies for each of those instances. Once you recognize the situations where you are most likely to smoke, you can work to avoid or change those situations as much as possible.

Remove Cigarettes and Other Tobacco Products

Stop purchasing cartons of cigarettes. Don't save any packs as souvenirs of your willpower to quit. Those extra packs of cigarettes only make it all too easy to start smoking again.

Take a look around you. Take note of all the visual cues that support your smoking so you can start eliminating them from your environment. For example, throw out ashtrays, lighters, and matches. Remove the lighter in your car. Clean your home, office, and car by using air freshener and ridding all remnants of cigarette smoke. Make an appointment with your dentist to have your teeth cleaned and polished. Try to avoid close contact with those who are smoking or carry the smell of smoke.

Talk to Your Health Care Provider

Make sure you discuss your quitting plan with your health care provider. If you are taking any prescription medications, find out how changing your smoking habits may affect your medications.

Nicotine is powerfully addictive. There are medications that can help you avoid withdrawal symptoms. Enlist the support of your health care provider, and discuss your options together.

Aids to Stop Smoking

Many products exist today to aid the transition to a smoke-free life. Studies show that people who use nicotine replacement therapy are almost twice as successful as those who do not. Some smoking-cessation aids are available over the counter; others require a prescription.

Nicotine Gum, Lozenges, and Patches

Nicotine gum, lozenges, and patches are available over the counter at your local pharmacy or grocery store. These products provide a low level of nicotine, without the accompanying toxins that come from smoking, to help you overcome the withdrawal symptoms.

The most common mistake people make with these products is not using enough. Do not skimp or underestimate the amount that you think that you will need. Follow the directions on the package, and do not forget to continue to use your product. Over time, you can reduce the amount you use. Always keep some of the medication around to help you avoid cravings. Different medications work better for different people. The main advantage of gum is it provides oral stimulation, just as cigarettes do. Patches allow a slower form of release over a longer period of time.

Nicotine Inhalers and Nasal Sprays

Nicotine inhalers and nasal sprays both require a prescription from your doctor. Nasal sprays can provide immediate relief. Furthermore, sprays come in different concentrations so you can reduce the amount of nicotine you put into your system over time.

Nicotine inhalers deliver nicotine into your system in much the same manner as cigarettes. For example, when you use a nicotine inhaler, you breathe the medication in through a mouthpiece. The nicotine is absorbed through the mouth's lining.

ESSENTIAL

When using an inhaler, gum, or lozenges, avoid eating or drinking acidic foods such as tomatoes, oranges, coffee, or soda within the first half hour of using the product—the acidic foods can neutralize the helpful effects of the product.

By using this inhalation technique, you best simulate the experience you had prior to quitting, allowing for an easier transition.

Bupropion

In contrast to the nicotine replacement therapies, bupropion pills, also known as Wellbutrin or Zyban, do not contain nicotine. Bupropion, originally developed as an antidepressant, was noticed to help reduce withdrawal symptoms and cigarette cravings. If you and your physician think this approach is good for you, you can even start taking the pill before your quit date.

This medication does require a prescription, however, and as it does have side effects, it is not appropriate for everyone. Medical experts recommend that pregnant women, people with eating disorders or who experience seizures, and people who drink heavily not use this medication.

Nicotine Poisoning

Take care not to smoke when you are using one of the nicotine replacement therapies. Keep in mind that these products are providing nicotine to your body and that it is possible to overdose, causing many symptoms due to the presence of nicotine receptors throughout your body. Know the signs of nicotine poisoning, which can include severe headaches, weakness, dizziness, nausea, vomiting, diarrhea, cold sweats, blurred vision, hearing difficulties, or mental confusion.

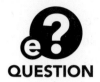

What should I do if I think I have nicotine poisoning?
Contact your health care provider or go to an emergency room if you experience any of the symptoms of nicotine poisoning when you are using a nicotine replacement product and you smoke. If you have any of these symptoms from wearing the patch, remove it immediately. Wash the surface of your skin with water.

After You Quit—Avoiding Relapse

Quitting the cigarette habit is among the most challenging tasks that you will face. Be prepared, particularly in the first few days and weeks, to have alternate plans to keep you busy and to help you avoid dwelling on your urges to have a cigarette. Those times of day when you are accustomed to sitting back and lighting up will require special preparation. Here are some suggestions for other ways to use this time:

- Take a walk.
- Allow yourself time for a nap.
- Have some healthy snacks around to chew on.
- Drink lots of water.
- Chew gum or suck on candy.
- Use breath spray.
- Perform breathing exercises.
- Hold something in your hand, like a pencil.
- Pick up a craft like knitting or crocheting to keep your hands busy.
- Exercise to reproduce the neurotransmitter stimulation.
- Enjoy a hot bath.
- Listen to music.
- Spend time with or call supportive friends.
- Buy yourself some fun magazines or a good book that you want to read.
- Visit public places where smoking is not allowed so that you cannot light up.

Certain pastimes are also best avoided in these first few critical weeks. To help you stay away from these triggers:

- Keep away from drinking alcoholic beverages.
- Limit caffeinated beverages, as too many can make you feel tense.
- Pass up invitations to spend time with people who smoke.
- If you must spend time with smokers, immediately inform them that you have quit.
- Practice refusing the offer of a cigarette so you will have your reply prepared.
- Steer clear of places where other people are smoking.
- Eat regularly, and include snacks to avoid extreme feelings of hunger.
- Surround yourself with supportive friends and family, and stay away from circumstances that inflame strong emotions such as anger, resentment, or loneliness.
- Avoid high-stress situations as much as possible.
- Try not to push yourself into feeling overly tired.
- Pamper and spoil yourself, and indulge in other pleasures.

When a strong smoking urge strikes, immediately engage in one of your alternate activities. If you find yourself daydreaming about smoking, turn your thoughts to another subject. Continue to remind yourself of all the great benefits that you will experience once you have quit your habit. Exercise and meditate to increase positive feelings and reduce stress. Post visual reminders—photos of loved ones, or whatever motivates you—to keep you on track with your goal.

If you do slip up, stop and forgive yourself. Get right back on your program. Remember that one cigarette is less harmful than an entire pack. Remind yourself that you can succeed and that you have strong reasons to quit.

Smoke-Free for Life

Nicotine can be as addicting as heroin, so give yourself plenty of pats on the back for quitting and staying smoke-free. It is quite an accomplishment, and you deserve a reward. One tangible way that you can reward yourself is to set aside a quit jar, where you put all the money you would normally have spent on your smoking habit. As often as you used to go out and buy a pack of cigarettes, put the money you would have used into your jar. After one month, take all the funds and indulge yourself by buying something purely for fun. Keep up this reward practice as long as you need that type of incentive and reminder to stay smoke-free.

FACT

Nicotine is a poison. If infants, children, or pets come into contact with or eat a nicotine patch, even a used one, it can cause serious harm. This is a medical emergency. If this occurs, contact your health care provider, emergency department, or poison control center immediately. Consider this another powerful reason to quit your habit as soon as possible.

Another critical factor is to follow the instructions of your nicotine replacement medication, if you are using one to assist you with quitting. A common mistake is for people to discontinue using the patch or gum a little sooner than recommended because they feel they have successfully overcome the urge to smoke. This can often lead to a relapse. Avoid this temptation. The first few months may remain challenging, so give yourself the extra support.

Another behavior that often leads to a relapse is the thought, "I'll just have one more. What can it hurt?" Studies show that even one more cigarette can often lead to a relapse and the need to repeat the difficult process of quitting. Remind yourself that the toughest time is those first few weeks, and that you do not want to go through the challenging process again. If it helps, write down the reasons you want to quit and post them in a visible place. Think about the health of yourself and others and the effects of your health on others.

Starting a new exercise program can often help to stay smoke-free. A walking program is not only easy, but it can also improve your health and allow you to enjoy the feeling of taking deep breaths and the smell of fresh air. Regular walking can also help with managing any extra weight gain that resulted from kicking the smoking habit. Exercise releases many of the same stimulants and neurotransmitters of smoking, making the quitting process easier. It also helps reduce stress, further reducing the temptation to light up. Other methods of reducing stress, such as meditation and relaxation, can similarly help reduce those urges.

Simply take a moment to truly acknowledge the power of your own convictions to create better health for yourself. You can be your best. Take each day one step at a time. Congratulate yourself for choosing health, not only for yourself, but also for your loved ones and everyone else who is around you.

CHAPTER 13

Drug Therapy for Cholesterol Management

Reducing your risk of cardiovascular disease, disability, and death requires that you make a commitment to support and enhance healthful living. Medications support this process. Drugs can be valuable tools to help you achieve optimal health. For some people, drug therapy to manage lipid levels is the best short-term action, until lifestyle changes have time to improve cardiovascular health. For others, drug therapy is the only way to address genetic tendencies toward unhealthy lipid levels.

When to Use Drugs to Treat High Cholesterol

This chapter provides an overview of the various drugs frequently prescribed to manage lipids, such as statins, bile acid sequestrants, nicotinic acid, and fibrates. These are the most common drugs prescribed to treat cholesterol, either alone or in combination. As you read about side effects, keep in mind that pharmaceuticals are potentially very beneficial. Do not become alarmed by precautions and necessary safeguards—it's important to have information to make intelligent choices. Medications, like most medical interventions, require an examination of the risk versus benefit. This is why medications are often considered only after lifestyle changes. While the side effects of medications are potentially harmful, the effects of most lifestyle changes, such as eating better, stopping smoking, exercising more, and decreasing stress, are only beneficial.

Studies show that drug therapy is more effective when used together with lifestyle changes to achieve healthy cholesterol levels and reduce the risk of heart attack and stroke. All therapies, therefore, require consideration in the context of your lifestyle.

When you incorporate a multipronged approach, you get results more quickly, you are able to reduce your medication levels sooner, and you will feel the improvements in your health more rapidly.

Statins, Your First Line of Defense

For physicians, statins are usually the drugs of choice for improving cholesterol levels. The primary goal of all lipid therapy is reduction of LDL cholesterol. Since statins lower LDL cholesterol more than any other type of drug while raising HDL and lowering triglycerdies, physicians typically consider statins first. Statins, like many lifestyle changes, improve all aspects of one's lipid profile and therefore have the most beneficial cardiovascular effect. Statins typically are the least prone to side effects of various medical therapies, despite still having significant potential effects.

Statins accomplish this reduction of LDL by blocking an enzyme, HMG-CoA reductase, which produces cholesterol in the liver. With this enzyme inhibited, the liver manufactures less cholesterol. Since the liver needs cholesterol, it removes more cholesterol from the bloodstream to replace what it is blocked from making. In this manner, statins reduce LDL production and also boost the body's ability to remove excess LDL cholesterol circulating in the bloodstream.

Statin Research Studies

Depending on the dosage, statins have shown the ability to reduce LDL levels up to 60 percent. A higher dosage is also associated with more significant side effects. Aggressive statin therapy has proved to reduce cardiac risk in very high-risk individuals by up to 60 percent and stroke risk by almost 20 percent.

Other large studies have shown that statin use decreased the risk of heart attack, stroke, peripheral arterial disease, and death in men and women, in middle-aged and older persons, and in people who had not yet had a heart attack as well as those who had survived a significant heart event. With results like these, physician confidence in the use of statins is high. They are generally considered a very cost-effective medication, second only to aspirin, in the prevention of heart attack and stroke.

Statin Types and Usage

Types of statins include but are not limited to lovastatin, simvastatin, pravastatin, fluvastatin, and atorvastatin. These are marketed under the brand names Mevacor, Zocor, Pravachol, Lescol, and Lipitor, respectively. Since the body makes more cholesterol at night than during the day, patients are usually directed to take statins in a single dose at the evening meal or at bedtime.

Typically, statins impact cholesterol levels the most by about four to six weeks. After about six to eight weeks, your health care provider will retest your cholesterol levels to determine the effectiveness of the statin therapy and whether the dose requires adjustment.

Side Effects of Statins

Most people do not have serious side effects when taking statins. Some people may experience constipation, stomach pain, cramps, or gas. These symptoms are usually mild to moderate, however, and they go away over time. More serious side effects can result from an increase in liver enzymes that can lead to liver toxicity. Because of this risk, it's important to have your liver function tested periodically while you are on statin therapy. People with active chronic liver disease should not take statins.

Another serious side effect comes from statin myopathy. Muscle soreness, pain, and weakness may occur. In extreme cases, muscle cells can break down and release the protein myoglobin into the blood. Myoglobin in the urine can contribute to impaired kidney function, eventually leading to kidney failure. The risk of this occurring increases when statins are taken at high dosages or combined with certain other cholesterol medications.

ALERT

Certain studies have shown a possible increased risk of amnesia and other memory-related problems while on statins. While this is possibly a rare side effect, more research is required. Since cholesterol is essential to cell membrane structure, scientists suggest that reducing cholesterol may affect neurological functioning.

Since statins affect the cell membrane's synthesis of cholesterol, women who are pregnant or planning to become pregnant should absolutely avoid them.

Avoid consuming grapefruit juice, grapefruits, or tangelos (a hybrid grapefruit) when you are taking statins, as these fruits can affect how the drug is metabolized. Grapefruits contain a chemical that affects certain digestive enzymes as drugs are broken down in the intestinal tract and liver. Interestingly, this effect can occur even if you wait twenty-four hours to take the medication. Therefore, if you are taking statins, it is best to avoid grapefruit products entirely.

Bile Acid Sequestrants or Resins

Bile acid sequestrants, also referred to as bile acid resins, reduce LDL cholesterol by binding with cholesterol-rich bile acids in the intestines to facilitate their elimination from the body through the stool. Think back to the liver's role in the cholesterol-manufacturing process. The liver uses cholesterol to manufacture bile acids, a digestive enzyme that breaks down fats. Bile acid sequestrants cause the body to eliminate bile acids in the intestines. Since the body needs bile acids to digest fats, the liver must manufacture more bile acids to replace those eliminated by the drug. The liver uses up its available cholesterol to make more acids, thus making less cholesterol available for release into the bloodstream. Bile acid sequestrants can reduce LDL cholesterol levels from 10 to 20 percent. Bile acid resins, however, can raise triglycerides.

Bile Acid Sequestrants Research Studies

Researchers have found a reduction in risk of coronary artery disease through the use of bile acid sequestrants, though this reduction is not nearly as significant as the risk reduction with statins.

Types of bile acid resins include cholestyramine (brand name Prevalite or Questran) and colestipol (Colestid). Cholestyramine and colestipol are often taken as powders that are mixed with water or fruit juice and taken either once or twice a day with meals. Both drugs are also available as tablets.

FACT

Federal government guidelines call for consideration of bile acid sequestrants as LDL-lowering therapy for women with elevated LDL cholesterol who are considering pregnancy, or for combination therapy with statins in people with very high LDL cholesterol levels.

Bile Acid Sequestrants Side Effects

The principal side effects with the use of bile acid resins have to do with digestion. This type of drug can cause a variety of gastrointestinal problems, such as constipation, bloating, fullness, nausea, abdominal pain, and gas. Drinking lots of water and eating high-fiber foods can help with these side effects. Physicians generally do not prescribe bile acid resins to people with a history of constipation problems.

Taking bile acids can also inhibit the absorption of certain nutrients from foods and of other medications. Physicians recommend that you take other prescription medications at least one hour before or at least four to six hours after the bile acid sequestrant. They also inhibit the absorption of fat-soluble vitamins from food, namely vitamins A, D, E, and K, so vitamin

supplementation is possibly necessary, especially if taking bile acid sequestrants during pregnancy.

Nicotinic Acid

Nicotinic acid, also known as niacin or vitamin B3, is gaining favor as a way
to reduce total blood cholesterol, LDL cholesterol, and triglyceride levels,
and to elevate HDL levels.

At extremely high doses, nicotinic acid raises HDL cholesterol and trans-
forms small LDL into the less harmful, normal-sized LDL cholesterol. Niacin
therapy moderately reduces LDL cholesterol levels. Among all the pharmaceutical choices, nicotinic acid is the most effective in raising HDL cholesterol.

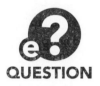

QUESTION

**Can you just take high doses of over-the-counter niacin for your
high cholesterol?**
Self-treatment with niacin is not safe. Since dosage and timing are important, people should not attempt to self-medicate with over-the-
counter B3 vitamins. Treatment with this medication should take place
only under the recommendation and supervision of a doctor.

Nicotinic Acid Research Studies

Studies demonstrate the power of niacin treatment on lipid disorders.
Patients treated with immediate-release niacin have seen their HDL levels
increase 15 to 35 percent, along with a 20 to 50 percent reduction in triglycerides and a 10 to 20 percent reduction in LDL cholesterol. Niacin has
been shown to help reverse atherosclerosis, therefore likely decreasing the
chance of a heart attack or stroke.

Nicotinic Acid Types and Usage

Niacin formulations come in three categories: immediate release, short-
term or intermediate release, and sustained or slow-acting release. If you are
a candidate for niacin therapy, your physician will determine what formula-

tion most suits you. Most physicians start patients on a low dose and work up to a daily dose of 1.5 to 3g. This improves the body's acceptance of the drug.

Another important consideration among different products is the quality of the niacin and the amount the body will absorb. A challenge with many over-the-counter supplements is they are prepared in forms that do not break down easily in the digestive system. They essentially pass through the body, without allowing for absorption of any nutrients. Supplements are not regulated by the U.S. Food and Drug Administration and are therefore not guaranteed to provide what is shown on the labels.

Niaspan, produced by KOS Pharmaceuticals, is specially formulated and packaged in a way that makes it clear how to regulate the levels of niacin in the bloodstream. Nicotinamide is another form of niacin; however, it is not effective in lowering cholesterol levels.

Nicotinic Acid Side Effects

The challenge with niacin treatment is tolerability. Flushing or hot flashes and itching, the result of the opening of blood vessels, are the most common side effects. If you titrate the drugs appropriately, however, the side effects should decrease over time as your body becomes more tolerant of the therapy. Taking niacin during or after meals and additional medications recommended by your physician can also decrease flushing. Taking aspirin thirty minutes prior to niacin has shown to reduce the incidence of flushing by 90 percent.

Federal government guidelines suggest nicotinic acid as a therapeutic option for higher-risk people, often as part of combination therapy, or as a single agent if the higher-risk person does not have high LDL cholesterol levels.

Other side effects include gastrointestinal upset such as nausea, indigestion, gas, vomiting, diarrhea, and even peptic ulcers. More serious risks include liver problems, gout, and high blood sugar. These risks increase as the dosage level is increased.

People who take high blood pressure medications also need to exercise caution with niacin therapy. Taking niacin can amplify the effects of blood pressure medications. People with diabetes typically do not receive niacin therapy because of its effect on blood sugar.

Fibrates

Physicians prescribe fibrates, or fibric acid derivatives, primarily to reduce triglycerides but also to increase HDL cholesterol. Fibrates, however, do not lower LDL cholesterol. Since LDL reduction is usually the primary target of therapy, fibrates are not typically physicians' drug of choice for individuals with elevated cholesterol levels. You should, however, evaluate the relevance of fibrate therapy to your individual case, since it is the drug of choice to reduce the most harmful small, dense LDL particles.

Fibrate therapy is a treatment option for people with coronary artery disease who have low LDL cholesterol but who still have unhealthy triglyceride levels. Physicians may prescribe fibrates along with statins for people who have both high levels of LDL cholesterol and unhealthy triglyceride levels.

Fibrate Research Studies

Studies show that fibrates can reduce triglycerides by as much as 20 to 50 percent and can increase HDL cholesterol by 10 to 15 percent. According to federal government guidelines, physicians can prescribe fibrates to people with very high triglycerides to reduce risk of acute pancreatitis, as extremely high triglyceride levels can occasionally cause inflammation of the pancreas.

Types of Fibrates and Usage

Gemfibrozil and fenofibrate are types of fibrates, known by the brand names Lopid and Tricor. Clofibrate is the third fibrate available in the United States. People on fibrate therapy typically take a dose twice daily, usually thirty minutes before their morning and evening meals.

Fibrate Side Effects

Most people do not suffer any adverse side effects from fibrate therapy. Some people, however, do experience gastrointestinal problems or headache, dizziness, blurred vision, runny nose, fatigue, or flushing. For some people, fibrates increase the chances of developing gallstones. Combining statins with fibrates may increase muscle cell breakdown, or rhabdomyolysis, which can potentially also harm the kidneys that receive the products of the muscle breakdown. Tell your health care provider right away about any side effects, particularly if you experience muscle or joint pain or weakness.

ALERT

Taking fibrates can increase the effect of blood-thinning medications. If you are taking both fibrates and blood thinners, work closely with your physician to monitor the effect of the fibrates.

Combination Drug Therapy

Your physician may prescribe combination drug therapy, depending on the characteristics of your lipid profile and whether you already have heart disease. The target LDL is more aggressive for people with certain existing problems. For people with existing heart disease or diabetes, the goal is to attain an LDL level of less than 100mg/dL or lower. To achieve this low level, your physician may prescribe a combination of LDL- and triglyceride-lowering medications, or a drug to elevate HDL levels, in addition to lifestyle changes. If you have two or more risk factors, but you do not have coronary artery disease or its equivalent, then the LDL target goal is to achieve an LDL level of less than 130mg/dL. This may also require combination drug therapy. For people who have one or no risk factors, but who do have elevated cholesterol levels, the target for LDL cholesterol is to achieve a level of less than 160mg/dL. Such an individual may require only LDL-lowering drugs. Depending on the combination of drugs, side effects may decrease due to needing a lower dosage of each drug, or increase due to drug interactions.

When you are put on therapeutic medications, your physician will regularly monitor your lipid levels to ascertain your progress. If you do not reach your goal after three months with a single drug, your doctor may recommend a second medicine to improve your progress. A combined drug approach may accelerate the lowering of your cholesterol. If you report particular side effects to your physician, he or she may also prescribe lower doses of a combination of medications to lessen the possibility of adverse effects.

Tips for Following Your Medication Program

Following your doctor's recommendations makes sense. Your health care provider is a trained professional who has taken time and effort to develop a program of therapy to support your well-being. Studies show that many patients do not follow medical advice. If you have taken the time to pursue a program of lipid-lowering medications, make the best of this support and follow your medication program. The following tips can help you.

FACT

According to the American Heart Association, 10 percent of all hospital admissions are patients who did not take their medications according to the instructions. The average stay in American hospitals due to medical noncompliance is 4.2 days. More than half of all Americans with chronic diseases do not follow their physician's medication and lifestyle instructions.

One of the most important things you can do to help you to stay on your medication program is to understand exactly what type of medication you are taking and why it is best for a person in your condition. This requires you to take some initiative to educate yourself about your lipid profile, your cholesterol goals, and your dosage schedule. Ask your health care provider the following questions:

- What is my lipid profile and what is the goal of my therapy?
- What type of medication (statin, nicotinic acid, fibrate) am I taking?
- Why is that medication best for a person in my condition?

- Are there any food/drug combinations I should avoid?
- When should I take the medicine and should I take it with, before, or after meals?
- What should I do if I forget to take a dose?
- What are the side effects of the medication and when should I contact a health care provider?
- Who should I contact, and how, in case I have negative side effects?

Consistency is essential to getting the most out of your therapeutic program. Do not change your dosage amount or schedule or quit taking prescription medications without consulting your physician. If you have a hard time with consistency, try some of the following tips:

- Take your medicine at the same time each day.
- Take your medicine when you perform a specific daily act, such as before you brush your teeth.
- Set your watch alarm as a pill reminder.
- Write yourself a note in a prominent place.
- Use a pillbox that holds each day's prescriptions in their respective compartments in a place where you will not forget to take them at the appropriate time.
- Write prescription renewal notes in your calendar to remind you before prescriptions run out.

If none of these tips help, consult with your pharmacist for more ideas. Work together with your health care provider as a team. Observe your reactions to the medication. Take notes, and report everything back to your physician. Keep your follow-up appointments so you can discuss how things are going. Bring your observation notes to your appointment to remind you of things you may easily forget. Bring your prescription bottles as well. Follow your progress from visit to visit—record data in a cholesterol-monitoring log. If you have questions, ask them; communication is critical to getting the best health care.

Natural Alternatives

There are numerous ways to naturally lower your cholesterol. Lifestyle changes are the most important natural therapy. As explained in previous chapters, the best ways to do this are by exercising more, stopping smoking, reducing stress, and improving your diet, including substituting foods high in saturated and trans fats with more plant-based foods rich in complex carbohydrates and a modest amount of unsaturated fats.

As with most prevalent medical issues, you will always find people who claim they have found breakthroughs to curing your cholesterol. Beyond many of the lifestyle changes discussed in this book, most of these are not scientifically proven remedies. Some suggested therapies include:

- Red Yeast Rice
- Garlic
- Coenzymes Q10
- Pantothine
- Gugulipid

While researchers have studied many of these to an extent and there is various literature supporting their use, none as yet is an officially recommended therapy.

Other nutritional supplement therapies aim to simulate the content in certain helpful foods that is considered the main source of their cholesterol profile benefits. These supplements include:

- Fish Oil
- Flax Seeds
- Plant Sterols and Stanols

While these may have more support as they are considered the key ingredients in certain foods that help your cholesterol profile, they also are yet to receive endorsement from any official guidelines or recommendations.

CHAPTER 14

Other Silent Killers

As noted earlier, people with diabetes are at higher risk for heart disease than those without. People who have high blood pressure are also at higher risk than those with normal blood pressure. People who have a cluster of metabolic disorders, characterized as the metabolic syndrome, are at a much greater risk for heart disease. Often, these diseases do not give any warning before they occur, and many people go for years without knowing they have them—and therefore without intervening. This chapter reviews some of these threatening silent killers in more detail and what you can do to address them.

Metabolic Disorders

Metabolic disorders occur when a specific enzyme or cofactor is absent or is present in insufficient quantities, which results in the body's inability to receive particular nutrients. In other words, the body is unable to metabolize foods into nutrients for fuel or to build tissue. For people who have problems producing insulin, which is the key to the uptake of blood glucose (blood sugar), the body is unable to use the glucose that is circulating in the bloodstream for fuel. As a result, blood-sugar levels become elevated.

If blood-glucose levels are elevated because insulin is not available or insulin resistance is severe, the person is diagnosed with diabetes, which is a metabolic disorder. If, on the other hand, blood-glucose levels are elevated because insulin sensitivity is impaired, and this impairment is present with other specific conditions, the person is considered to have a metabolic disorder, described as the "metabolic syndrome." Both of these conditions increase the risk of heart disease. Many people with diabetes, including children and adults, also have lipid disorders, and many also have hypertension. Both of these conditions increase the risk of heart disease. Therefore, people with diabetes not only need to manage their blood sugar, but it is also important for them to manage their blood pressure and cholesterol carefully.

What Is Hypertension?

Those who have high blood pressure are said to have hypertension. Pressure equals the force of something over a certain area. In the case of the blood pressure, the force is exerted by blood vessels on vessel walls. When this pressure is elevated, the walls become thickened and less elastic, with greater damage to the vessel walls. The increased pressure also means the heart has to pump blood with a greater force. All of these changes put you at higher risk for cardiovascular disease.

Blood pressure has two values shown as an upper number and a lower number. The upper number represents the "systolic" blood pressure, or the greater pressure exerted by the heart and blood when the heart is pumping. The lower number, the "diastolic" pressure, represents the pressure of the blood when the heart is relaxed.

The pressure is measured in millimeters of mercury, also written as mmHg (Hg is the abbreviation for mercury on the periodic table). The threshold for elevated blood pressure is 140(systolic)/90(diastolic) mmHg. Having a systolic or diastolic blood pressure greater than these values on repeated manual checks will often result in a diagnosis of hypertension. Like cholesterol, blood pressure will often respond to lifestyle changes, so that remains first-line therapy. If the blood pressure is resistant to such changes, then there are myriad medications to treat high blood pressure.

ALERT

High blood pressure is one of the most prevalent diseases in society, and its prevalence increases as our population ages because blood pressure gets higher as we get older. Because of its prevalence and the harm it can cause when unrecognized, decreasing high blood pressure is one of the most effective preventative measures you have for reducing cardiovascular disease.

Over the past two decades, more attention has been focused on those whose high blood pressure is in a "borderline" zone of above 120/90 mmHg but below the threshold for hypertension. These people are now labeled "prehypertensives." Like those whose cholesterol is in a borderline zone, these people often get checked more frequently and are encouraged to make lifestyle changes before becoming hypertensive. If there are multiple other cardiovascular risk factors, pharmaceutical treatment may start, as there apparently is some benefit even from escaping this prehypertensive zone.

What Is Diabetes?

When you eat foods that are rich in carbohydrates, such as breads, cereals, or grains, your body breaks it down into glucose. Also referred to as blood sugar, your body can use glucose for energy. In a normally functioning system, a healthy pancreas releases insulin into the bloodstream, and this insulin helps to remove the glucose from your bloodstream for your cells to use as fuel. In people who have diabetes, this process is dysfunctional. Either their bodies do not produce any insulin, or the insulin they produce cannot be used.

Because their bodies cannot convert the sugar in the blood into energy, people with diabetes have high levels of glucose in their bloodstream. The kidneys of diabetic people need to work extra hard to filter the blood to remove the excess glucose. This causes frequent urination and excessive thirst from fluid loss.

FACT

Diabetes can lead to many dangerous conditions, particularly if untreated or incorrectly managed. These include heart disease, stroke, kidney disease and kidney failure, nerve damage, and gum disease. The disease also raises the risk threefold of dying from complications related to influenza or pneumonia. In America, diabetes is currently the sixth-leading cause of death and is a leading cause of blindness and amputations.

The liver is also involved in the process of maintaining normal blood-sugar levels. After you eat, the sugars from the food enter your bloodstream and are available as fuel, along with the triglycerides. If not all the sugar fuel is used, either due to poor processing based on low insulin or a reduced need for energy based on a low activity level, the liver removes the excess sugar from the bloodstream, much in the same manner as it removes excess cholesterol, and stores it in the liver as glycogen. If for some reason you are unable to eat, the liver later can release this stored glucose into the bloodstream to provide an energy boost. This helps to keep your blood-sugar levels in a more constant range.

Diabetes consists of two main types, both characterized by the body's inability to process available sugar into energy. The two major types are Type 1 and Type 2 diabetes. People with either type can experience elevated blood-glucose levels.

Type 1 Diabetes

Type 1 diabetes is an autoimmune condition that occurs most often in children and adults younger than age thirty. It is also called juvenile-onset diabetes or insulin-dependent diabetes mellitus. This condition occurs when the body does not produce any insulin, so people with this type of diabetes take daily insulin injections. Approximately 5 to 10 percent of people with diabetes have Type 1. Young people with diabetes are not likely to have heart disease in their youth. As they age, however, their risk of heart disease is greater than the risk for those who do not have diabetes.

Type 2 Diabetes

Type 2 is the most common form of diabetes. It affects about 90 to 95 percent of people who have diabetes. This type of diabetes is referred to as maturity-onset diabetes, adult-onset diabetes, or non–insulin-dependent diabetes mellitus.

Type 2 diabetes is a metabolic disorder. In this case, the pancreas produces some insulin but not enough to allow the sugar to enter the body's cells. At the same time, muscle and tissue cells develop a resistance to the insulin. Therefore, even though sugar is flowing in the bloodstream, the body's tissues remain "hungry." Scientists are still unable to identify the exact mechanism for why insulin resistance occurs, but it seems to have a relationship to excess body fat.

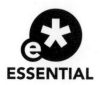

ESSENTIAL

Your risk of heart disease increases regardless of whether you have Type 1 or Type 2 diabetes. People with Type 1 diabetes are unlikely to get heart disease when they are young, yet as they grow older, their risk becomes higher than the risk of their peers without diabetes.

The Relationship Between Diabetes, Hypertension, and Heart Disease

When a person has diabetes or hypertension, he or she is also more likely to develop heart disease. Depending on the diabetic's or hypertensive's number of risk factors, the person may face an even greater risk of heart disease. For example, someone who has diabetes, high blood pressure, high cholesterol, who smokes, and who is completely inactive is at far greater risk of heart disease than someone who only has diabetes. Therefore, controlling risk factors that you can change is extremely important in improving overall health.

ESSENTIAL

Diabetes increases a woman's risk of heart disease by three to seven times, compared with a two- to threefold increase in risk for men, according to the American Heart Association. While it is important for all people with diabetes to take extra good care of their health, this is even more necessary for women.

Scientists believe that diabetes increases your risk of heart disease because persistent elevated levels of blood sugar damages arteries. If you recall how atherosclerotic plaque gets started, you will remember that plaque begins to form on areas where the inside lining of the blood vessels is damaged. Scientists continue to research other mechanisms to explain why people with diabetes are at such an increased risk of heart disease.

Getting Tested for Diabetes

You can determine whether you have diabetes by having the levels of glucose in the bloodstream measured. Before you take a test for diabetes, it is recommended that you go without anything but water for at least nine to twelve hours, as when getting your cholesterol tested.

ALERT

"Prediabetes," or impaired fasting glucose, is a condition characterized by higher-than-normal blood-glucose levels that are not high enough for diagnosis as Type 2 diabetes. The American Diabetes Association (ADA) estimates that almost 20 million Americans have prediabetes. If you have this condition, work with your physician right away to start taking steps to lower your blood-sugar levels.

A normal result for a fasting glucose test is between 65 and 109mg/dL. A result that is between 110 to 125mg/dL could indicate an impaired fasting glucose level, also known as prediabetes. Like prehypertension, this may require more frequent monitoring or lifestyle changes. A result that is higher than 126mg/dL could indicate diabetes.

Signs and Symptoms of Diabetes

People often disregard the symptoms of diabetes. However, studies indicate that if diabetes is detected early, people can reduce the likelihood that complications will develop. Therefore, it is important to know the signs and symptoms of diabetes, particularly if you have a family history of this disease. The signs and symptoms of diabetes include the following:

- Frequent urination
- Excessive thirst
- Extreme hunger
- Unusual weight loss
- Increased fatigue
- Irritability
- Numbness or tingling in feet or legs
- Slow-healing cuts or bruises
- Blurry vision

Types of Tests

To test your blood-glucose levels, you can either have a finger-prick fasting blood sugar test, or you can have a hemoglobin A1C test. The tests differ in that a finger-prick test provides a measure of your blood sugar at the moment of the test, while the hemoglobin A1C test shows the regulation of your blood sugar over the past three-month period by analyzing the hemoglobin, instead of simply the sugar levels. In order to establish a diagnosis of diabetes, a hemoglobin A1C test is necessary.

The American Diabetes Association recommends that people with diabetes take the hemoglobin A1C test two to four times a year. The hemoglobin A1C test does not replace daily self-testing but rather provides a method to assess your success with blood sugar management over time. The U.S. Food and Drug Administration has approved a home test. Check with your health care provider to see if it is appropriate for you.

FACT

Approximately 1 million people are diagnosed with diabetes every year. The percentage of American adults with diagnosed diabetes, including women with a history of gestational diabetes (diabetes during pregnancy), has soared over the past two decades. Minority racial and ethnic populations are particularly at risk of developing the disease.

Testing Tips

Fortunately, getting tested for diabetes and high blood pressure is quite easy. Oftentimes workplaces or health fairs will put on health screenings that will check your blood pressure and blood sugar for free. As with cholesterol, to get a true blood sugar measurement you should fast for at least nine hours prior to getting tested, as meals or many drinks will falsely elevate your blood sugar. Even salty meals can temporarily elevate your blood pressure, as can nervousness or going through normal bodily cycles based on the time of day.

Make sure to get repeated checks, ideally by your health care provider, before establishing a diagnosis of diabetes or hypertension. These screenings are meant to increase awareness regarding yourself and the disease in general. If during these screenings your blood pressure or sugar is elevated, you should consult with your health care provider. Do this promptly, but not necessarily emergently. Remember, diabetes and hypertension are silent killers. This means they linger for years and years harming your body. Having high blood pressure or sugar for a day, week, month, or even longer is not necessarily that harmful. However, carrying these risks for years will do you harm.

What You Can Do

If your doctor diagnoses you with diabetes or hypertension, it's even more important that you adopt healthy lifestyle habits. When you address the root causes of this condition—excess weight, a sedentary lifestyle, and diet—sensitivity to insulin is restored, and the risk factors are reduced. Lifestyle changes can make a huge difference. If you have diabetes or hypertension, you can successfully manage it. If you are prediabetic, you can avoid becoming diabetic. If you are prehypertensive, you can avoid becoming hypertensive.

The Power of Healthful Eating

Physical activity and healthful eating need to go together to improve the factors associated with diabetes and the metabolic syndrome. Healthy nutrition should follow the guidelines discussed in Chapter 8, including eating a diet of primarily plant-based foods. Total dietary fat should represent no more than 25 to 35 percent of total calories, and it should consist almost entirely of unsaturated vegetable fats. Researchers note that dietary fat, rather than calories, carbohydrates, or even sugar intake, is seemingly a critical factor in Type 2 diabetes, although they have not yet identified the exact mechanisms. Losing weight improves blood pressure as well. Decreasing salt intake with each meal will decrease blood pressure on a daily basis.

The Power of Exercise

Your exercise program to improve insulin sensitivity should include both heart-pumping cardiovascular activities and strength-training exercises to tone up your muscles. Regular exercise helps you maintain healthy blood-sugar levels by burning fuels and by helping you to achieve and maintain a healthy weight and shed excess body fat. Improvements in glucose tolerance and insulin sensitivity are usually short-lived, however, and deteriorate within three days of your last workout. This factor makes regular aerobic exercise vital. Exercise also promotes reductions in blood pressure by creating new blood vessels, thereby causing less pressure, thickening, and damage to individual vessels. It also makes your heart stronger and better able to pump.

Cardiovascular or aerobic exercise, such as walking, is critically important for lowering blood pressure, managing blood-sugar levels, and improving your body's ability to use insulin. Try to be active on at least three nonconsecutive days and up to five sessions per week. Ideally, your aerobic exercise session should last at least thirty minutes. It's not necessary to work at a high intensity. Take it easy, and progress gradually. If thirty minutes is too long, start with ten-minute bouts and accumulate thirty minutes in one day.

According to the position taken by the American College of Sports Medicine (ACSM) on exercise and Type 2 diabetes, resistance or weight training has the potential to improve muscle strength and endurance, enhance flexibility and body composition, decrease risk factors for cardiovascular disease, and result in improved glucose tolerance and insulin sensitivity. Strength training can also increase the resting metabolic rate to assist in weight control. Regular exercise that includes aerobics and strength training also provides important emotional health benefits, including reduced stress, heightened feelings of well-being, and enhanced quality of life.

Exercise Risks for People with Diabetes and Hypertension

Before you begin your exercise program, consult with your health care provider, as exercise affects blood-sugar levels and blood pressure. Exercise helps to decrease blood-glucose concentrations, potentially reducing or eliminating insulin doses, especially for those with Type 2 diabetes. Exercise may also decrease or eliminate the need for blood pressure medications. You need to have a clear understanding of how activity and medications affect your blood-glucose levels to ensure your physical-activity program is both safe and effective.

Low Blood Sugar

The greatest exercise risk to people with diabetes is hypoglycemia, or low blood-sugar levels due the medications for diabetes. Hypoglycemia can lead to a life-threatening loss of consciousness. People with Type 2 diabetes that is controlled by meal planning and exercise usually do not have problems with low blood sugar. However, people who take insulin or oral diabetes medicine may have low blood-sugar levels both during and after exercise.

The risk of developing low blood glucose is greatest after high-intensity or extended exercise. This reaction can take place even twelve or more hours after a workout. To help prevent hypoglycemia, you must time your medications carefully. The ACSM recommends injecting insulin at least one hour before exercise. In addition, you need to ensure adequate food intake and monitor blood-glucose levels before and after exercise, as well as during longer exercise sessions or when trying a new activity.

The signs and symptoms of hypoglycemia include extreme fatigue, excessive sweating, headache, trembling, weakness, slurred speech, poor coordination, feeling faint, pale moist skin, full rapid pulse, and elevated blood pressure. If not dealt with, hypoglycemia can result in loss of consciousness or seizures.

ALERT

If you begin to experience hypoglycemia, you need to consume a rapidly absorbed sugar source immediately, such as a half cup of fruit juice or regular soda, two teaspoons of sugar or raisins, or six jelly beans or a piece of hard candy. To stay on the safe side, always keep a source of rapidly acting carbohydrate easily available during exercise and tell others where this source is located.

Since exercise burns fuel, you need to monitor food intake carefully in relationship to increased activity. ADA advises individuals with diabetes to exercise from one to three hours after eating a meal. One hour of exercise generally requires 15 additional grams of carbohydrates, which you should consume before or after exercise, depending on your individual condition and needs. If exercise is vigorous or longer than one hour, an additional 15 to 30g of carbohydrates are recommended for each additional hour.

Low Blood Pressure

Blood pressure medications act by lowering blood pressure, of course. In terms of your cardiovascular health, this can be a good thing. For exercise, this may be highly limiting. By lowering blood pressure, the body's ability to adequately meet the demand of strained organs becomes more challenging. Certain blood pressure medications act by decreasing the heart's rate and power of pumping. During exercise, though, the heart needs to beat faster and harder to adequately pump blood to exercising muscles. By decreasing blood pressure, all blood pressure medications, even ones that do not act directly on the heart, decrease the pressure of blood acting on your muscles. Again, during normal life this reduces your normal cardiovascular risk, but during exercise this decreases your ability to reach your maximum exercise capacity.

The effects of blood pressure and diabetes medicines on your ability to exercise represent a challenge. Blood pressure and sugar medicines decrease your cardiovascular risk. Exercise also reduces blood pressure and blood sugar as well as other cardiovascular risk factors. However, blood pressure and diabetes medications may reduce the ability to exercise. In other words, blood pressure and diabetes medications come with benefits and risks. These benefits and risks are dependent on your blood pressure or sugar, your ability to exercise and desire to exercise, and to what extent you can exercise. Only you and your health care provider can ultimately evaluate the risks versus benefits.

Dehydration

High blood-sugar levels can increase urination, contributing to dehydration. In addition, diabetic complications such as autonomic neuropathy, which affects the nerves serving internal organs and regulating blood pressure, blood glucose, and perspiration, may impair your sweating response, increasing the risk of heat-related illness. Certain blood pressure medications, called diuretics, work by increasing urination, decreasing the total amount of fluid coursing through your blood vessels, thereby decreasing pressure.

Make sure you drink fluids before, during, and after exercise, especially in warmer environments. Plain water is usually sufficient for sessions of one hour or less. Workouts lasting longer than one hour require water and extra carbohydrates. People with diabetes will absorb beverages with a 6 to 8 percent carbohydrate solution, such as sports drinks, more easily than soft drinks or fruit juices, which are typically 13 to 14 percent carbohydrate solutions.

Problems Due to Poor Circulation

People with diabetes need to protect their feet when they exercise. If you have a more severe case of diabetes with other risk factors such as hypertension, you may also have nerve damage or circulatory disorders, such as peripheral vascular disease. This may cause impaired blood flow to the extremities (the hands and feet). Extra protection of your feet will help prevent bruising or injury.

Wear appropriate athletic footwear, and wash and dry your feet thoroughly after exercising and check for sores. Petroleum jelly may help to decrease friction on specific areas. If you have an open sore that is not healing, consult a health care professional immediately. When not treated promptly, an infection can spread to the bone, resulting in amputation.

ALERT

Diabetes increases the risk for injuries to the feet in multiple ways. In addition to increasing atherosclerosis, which obstructs blood flow to the feet, diabetes can also decrease nerve sensation. This impairs one's ability to detect harmful lesions to the feet early when they are more treatable. In addition, because of poor blood flow, wounds tend to not heal as readily.

Avoid fitness equipment that may impair circulation, such as bands or buoyancy equipment on legs or feet in water exercise. Inadequate blood supply can make you more prone to pain, aching, or cramping during exercise. Rest for about two minutes if cramping occurs during a workout.

While it may seem as though there are a lot of precautions related to exercise, it is one of the best things you can do to help improve blood-sugar levels and insulin sensitivity. With a regular activity program and improved nutritional habits, you can avoid or control Type 2 diabetes. Regular exercise and healthy eating habits are also keys to weight management. With time and consistency, you can lose excess weight, restore insulin sensitivity, lower blood pressure, and reduce cholesterol and triglyceride levels. This may even make the use of further medications unnecessary.

CHAPTER 15

Special Groups and High Cholesterol

While the same general principles related to healthy nutrition, regular physical activity, no smoking, and weight and stress management apply to all people, there are certain special considerations for people with particular needs. These people include children, teens, and older adults. Women also have needs and special considerations distinct from those of men.

High Cholesterol in Children and Adolescents

Recently, medical professionals have started paying greater attention to childhood cholesterol levels as concerns rise over the increasing incidence of Type 2 diabetes, inactivity, and overweight issues among kids. Since heart disease is a slow, progressive disease, the significance of healthy habits in youth is gaining more and more attention.

An Inherited Disorder

Children from certain families that include a parent or grandparent who had heart disease at an early age are genetically prone to have high cholesterol levels. If a male relative had a heart attack before age fifty-five or a female relative before age sixty-five, this places a child in a high-risk category.

Statistics reveal that approximately one in 500 children have inherited hypercholesterolemia, or extremely high cholesterol levels. These children have a 50 percent risk of having heart disease before age fifty. If this condition is detected early, children can start incorporating healthy habits to greatly reduce their risk of having heart disease as adults.

Research has found fatty streaks that represent the beginning of atherosclerotic plaque in children as young as age three. Among children, girls tend to have higher total cholesterol and LDL levels than boys.

FACT

If you have a child with high cholesterol, take time to educate him or her about the value of healthy habits. Try not to portray the condition as a horrible disease. All kids and parents benefit from eating good foods and staying active. It's unnecessary for your child to feel stigmatized or to feel high levels of stress over the condition.

Guidelines for Blood Lipid Levels

The National Cholesterol Education Program's Expert Panel on Blood Cholesterol in Children and Adolescents recommends certain guidelines for cholesterol levels in children and adolescents age two to nineteen. According to these guidelines, total cholesterol is acceptable if it is less than 170mg/dL.

It is considered borderline if it is 170 to 199mg/dL and high if it is 200mg/dL or greater. Ideal LDL cholesterol is less than 110mg/dL, with borderline levels ranging from 110 to 129mg/dL. At levels of 130 or greater, LDL is considered high. The guidelines also recommend HDL levels of greater than or equal to 35mg/dL and triglycerides of less than or equal to 150mg/dL.

American children have much higher blood-cholesterol levels than children from other countries. The principal culprit is not genetics but poor nutrition, followed by lack of exercise. American kids typically eat a diet filled with highly processed fast foods rich in saturated fats, trans fats, and sugar.

ESSENTIAL

Direct role modeling is one of the most powerful ways to improve lifestyle habits of kids and teens. Help your children to have a healthy and disease-free adulthood by incorporating healthy lifestyle habits for the whole family. Plan physical activities together such as hiking or bike riding and keep healthy foods around the house.

Government treatment guidelines for children recommend lifestyle changes as the first line of therapeutic intervention. Improving eating habits, increasing physical activity, and managing weight can go a long way toward reducing elevated cholesterol levels. Certainly, these lifestyle habits are beneficial for all children, even those who are not from high-risk families.

Experts disagree about the role of cholesterol-lowering drugs for children. The American Heart Association and the federal government recommend considering cholesterol-lowering drugs only for those children over ten years of age who have high LDL levels even after changes in diet and activity. Other experts, however, remain concerned about the long-term effectiveness of drug therapy. Medical professionals uniformly believe healthful lifestyle changes are of paramount importance for children to enjoy good health.

Special Considerations for Teens

Teens, their parents, and health care providers also need to be sensitive to cholesterol issues affecting today's youth. Studies show that between 15 and 20 percent of the population already has atherosclerotic plaque by age twenty. These plaques lead to the cascade of blood vessel damage causing further plaque build-up that eventually leads to cardiovascular disease. Therefore, managing cholesterol in these early years can have a significant impact on later years. About 10 percent of adolescents between the ages of twelve to nineteen have cholesterol levels that exceed 200mg/dL.

This does not mean most young adults should be placed on cholesterol medications, though this may rarely be warranted. Instead, focus on lifestyle is extremely important. Because heart disease does not typically manifest during one's early years, there's a tendency to not consider the importance of a heart-healthy lifestyle. In addition, most teenagers often have a feeling of "being invincible," as though they can live any type of lifestyle without the lifestyle catching up to them.

Young adults are often indiscriminate in their diet. Busy parents are often lucky to find time in their child's or their own schedule, so quick foods are often eaten on the go. These quick foods are often heavily processed and laden with fat, salt, and simple carbohydrates. Schools, in an effort to cut costs, often serve food lacking in nutrition as well, though there's a significant movement to try to change this practice.

Finally, if not compelled to, many teens may choose to not participate in a regular exercise program, leading to excess weight and cholesterol levels. Schools provide less regular physical education than in previous decades, and young adults these days have the option of sitting at home on the computer rather than playing outside.

Using oral contraceptives and cigarettes further increases the risk for adolescents. In one study among females aged twelve to seventeen years, researchers found that the total cholesterol of oral contraceptive users was significantly higher than in nonusers. Birth control users who are also smokers are at even higher risk for heart disease.

Women with High Cholesterol

Heart disease is the number-one killer of women. In America, heart diseases kill nearly half a million women per year, more than the next seven causes of death, including all forms of cancer. The recommended levels of blood cholesterol are for the most part the same for women and men; however, women have some distinct differences that merit special consideration.

Other Concerns for Women

Pregnancy is a time in life when a woman's cholesterol profile tends to change. Pregnant women typically have an increase in blood-cholesterol levels. This is not cause for undue alarm, unless otherwise noted by your health care provider.

As mentioned previously, oral contraception can increase levels of blood cholesterol as well as blood pressure. Therefore, if you are taking birth control pills, it is even more important to engage in other health-enhancing practices. Smokers, in particular, have a higher risk of heart disease and stroke if they also take birth control pills.

Women may have a greater tendency to have atypical chest pain or to complain of abdominal pain, difficulty breathing, nausea, and unexplained fatigue. Also, although women are often known for urging their husbands or children to see the doctor, they tend to avoid or delay seeking medical care for themselves.

One more confounding factor in the diagnosis and treatment of heart disease in women is that diagnostic tests and procedures are not as accurate for women as they are for men. For example, an exercise stress test has a higher likelihood of showing a false positive or a false negative for women subjects.

The Age Factor: Cholesterol and Menopause

A woman's risk of heart disease increases approximately ten to fifteen years later than the average man's. This disparity is reflected in guidelines that state an age of forty-five or above is a risk factor for a man; for a woman, on the other hand, age does not become a risk factor until she is fifty-five. The reasons for this difference are not fully understood. Some of it is believed to be due to the protective effects of estrogen. A woman's heart disease risk rises when she becomes postmenopausal, regardless of whether menopause occurred naturally or as the result of surgery. Hormone replacement therapy, once hoped to decrease this risk, has not proved to do so.

By the time a woman reaches the age of seventy-five or older, her risk of heart attack is approximately the same as that of a man's. Women age seventy-five and above actually have a higher risk of death by stroke than men. The reasons for this are not clear. Some researchers suggest that it may simply stem from the fact that atherosclerosis is a slow, progressive disease and more women live longer than men. More research on women's health issues is needed to bring further light to these questions.

ALERT

Treatment of postmenopausal women with hormone replacement therapy was once theorized to reduce the heart disease risk in women; however, studies demonstrated that this hypothesis was incorrect. Medical experts no longer recommend estrogen treatment to prevent heart disease.

Another aspect of menopause that may contribute to a woman's higher risk of heart disease is the tendency to gain weight, particularly around the abdominal area. Abdominal fat that creates an apple-shaped physique is a known sign for increased risk of heart disease. While healthy habits are valuable throughout life, postmenopausal women should pay particular care to healthy nutrition and exercise habits, as well as to effective weight management.

Older Adults with High Cholesterol

Most deaths from heart disease occur in the older adult population. Men aged sixty-five and above and women aged seventy-five and above are classified as older adults for the purpose of discussing heart disease. Cholesterol levels, even in older age, have predictive power for the increased risk of heart disease. Furthermore, studies have shown that reducing LDL cholesterol levels also reduces the risk of death from heart disease. Therefore, maintaining healthy lifestyle habits is still valuable, even in older age.

Numerous therapies have proved significantly effective, no matter at what age they are implemented. Life extension can even occur at older ages. Quality of life is also important and is maintainable through healthy nutrition, regular physical activity, and weight management. Studies of people even over the age of ninety showed that strength training with weights could bring improvements.

A lifetime of healthy habits is always the ideal situation. But few people live ideal lives. Everyone can make daily life more pleasurable by enhancing health, which includes maintaining healthy lipid levels. It is never too late to take steps to improve the quality of daily living. So get started!

d Olives

rt-healthy oil.
ake.

small bowl, combine 2
oil and 1 tablespoon lemon
ture on both sides of the
sheet and bake for 10
ake for another 10–15
toasted. Remove from oven

r food processor, combine
olive oil, remaining 2
, the egg white, and mustard,
til blended and thick.

redients, cover, and refrigerate
e spread with the toasted

turated fat: 1.65g | Dietary fiber:
terol: 1.62mg

petizer,
es

Lemon Bruschetta with Choppe

Olives are high in sodium, but they contain a lot of he
This elegant appetizer is quick and easy to m

INGREDIENTS | SERVES 12

6 tablespoons olive oil

3 tablespoons lemon juice, divided

12 slices Three-Grain French Bread
(Chapter 19)

1 pasteurized egg white

2 tablespoons Dijon mustard

10 large black olives, chopped

10 large cracked green olives, chopped

½ cup chopped flat-leaf parsley

1 tablespoon fresh oregano leaves

¼ teaspoon crushed red pepper flakes

½ cup chopped toasted walnuts

1. Preheat oven to 375°F. I
   tablespoons of the olive
   juice, and brush this mi
   bread. Place on a cooki
   minutes, then turn and
   minutes or until bread i
   and cool on wire rack.

2. Meanwhile, in blender c
   remaining 4 tablespoon
   tablespoons lemon juice
   and blend or process ui

3. Stir in the remaining in§
   for 1 hour. Serve the oli·
   bread.

CALORIES: 200.09 | Fat: 11.94g | S
2.88g | Sodium: 152.59mg | Chole·

Super-Spicy Salsa

You can use salsa in so many ways. It's wonderful in frittatas and delicious as a garnish for chili or grilled chicken.

INGREDIENTS | YIELDS 3 CUPS; SERVING SIZE ¼ CUP

2 jalapeño peppers, minced
1 habanero pepper, minced
1 green bell pepper, minced
4 cloves garlic, minced
1 red onion, chopped
5 ripe tomatoes, chopped
3 tablespoons lemon juice
¼ teaspoon salt
⅛ teaspoon white pepper
¼ cup chopped fresh cilantro

1. In large bowl, combine jalapeños, habanero pepper, bell pepper, garlic, red onion, and tomatoes. In small bowl, combine lemon juice, salt, and pepper; stir to dissolve salt. Add to tomato mixture along with cilantro.

2. Cover and refrigerate for 3–4 hours before serving.

CALORIES: 25.23 | Fat: 0.21g | Saturated fat: 0.05g | Dietary fiber: 1.44g | Sodium: 53.25mg | Cholesterol: 0.0mg

Cucumber Dill Canapés

This cool, crisp, and creamy appetizer is very simple to make. If you pipe the cream cheese mixture on the cucumbers, it's suitable for a fancy party.

INGREDIENTS | SERVES 6

1 English cucumber
1 3-ounce package low-fat cream cheese, softened
1 tablespoon lemon juice
¼ cup nonfat whipped salad dressing
1 tablespoon minced fresh dill weed
Pinch white pepper

1. Wash cucumber and slice into ¼" slices. Arrange on a serving platter. In a small bowl, combine cream cheese with lemon juice and beat well. Add salad dressing, dill, and pepper and beat until smooth.

2. Spoon or pipe cream cheese mixture on cucumber slices. Serve immediately or cover and chill up to 4 hours before serving.

CALORIES: 80.23 | Fat: 5.94g | Saturated fat: 2.09g | Dietary fiber: 0.34g | Sodium: 114.68mg | Cholesterol: 7.94mg

English Cucumbers

Cucumbers are very high in water content and vitamin C. The skins of regular cucumbers are usually waxed; English cucumbers are not. You can serve them with the peel, which increases the fiber content. A component of cucumbers may help lower blood pressure.

Stuffed Jalapeño Peppers

These little peppers are super spicy. Serve them at the beginning of a Mexican meal.

INGREDIENTS | SERVES 6

12 small jalapeños

1 3-ounce package low-fat cream cheese, softened

1 tablespoon lemon juice

¼ cup Super-Spicy Salsa (see previous page)

1 teaspoon chopped fresh oregano

Working with Hot Peppers

Capsaicin is the ingredient that gives peppers their heat; it's also an ingredient in pepper spray! Use gloves when working with peppers and never, ever touch your face, especially your eyes, until you have removed the gloves and thoroughly washed your hands.

1. Cut jalapeños in half lengthwise. For a milder taste, remove membranes and seeds. Set aside.

2. In a small bowl, combine cream cheese with lemon juice; beat until fluffy. Add salsa and oregano and mix well.

3. Using a small spoon, fill each jalapeño half with the cream cheese mixture. Serve immediately or cover and chill for up to 8 hours before serving.

CALORIES: 45.98 | Fat: 2.70g | Saturated fat: 1.60g | Dietary fiber: 1.03g | Sodium: 51.15mg | Cholesterol: 7.94mg

Grilled Cherry Tomatoes with Parmesan Cheese

When cherry tomatoes are grilled, their flavor is intensified.
Each little tomato will burst with flavor in your mouth.

INGREDIENTS | SERVES 6

24 cherry tomatoes

1 tablespoon extra-virgin olive oil

1 tablespoon red-wine vinegar

⅛ teaspoon salt

Pinch white pepper

1 tablespoon chopped fresh mint

2 tablespoons shaved Parmesan cheese

1. Tear off an 18" × 12" sheet of heavy-duty aluminum foil. Poke cherry tomatoes with the tip of a knife and arrange on foil. In small bowl, combine oil, vinegar, salt, and pepper and mix well. Spoon over tomatoes.

2. Bring together foil edges and fold over several times, sealing the package. Leave some room for expansion.

3. Prepare and preheat grill. Grill the foil packet over medium coals for 4–6 minutes or until tomatoes are hot. Remove from grill, open package, and sprinkle with mint and shaved Parmesan. Serve immediately.

CALORIES: 43.92 | Fat: 3.78g | Saturated fat: 0.69g | Dietary fiber: 0.82g | Sodium: 107.03mg | Cholesterol: 1.33mg

Hawaiian Chicken Skewers

Serve these little skewers before a cookout featuring grilled hamburgers or turkey burgers and potato salad.

INGREDIENTS | SERVES 8

¼ cup coconut milk

1 tablespoon toasted sesame oil

½ teaspoon Tabasco sauce

¼ cup pineapple juice

1 pound chicken tenders

½ fresh pineapple, cut into chunks

2 tablespoons lime juice

1. In medium bowl, combine coconut milk, sesame oil, Tabasco sauce, and pineapple juice. Cut chicken crosswise and add to coconut milk mixture. Cover and refrigerate for 8 hours.

2. Alternate chicken pieces and pineapple on skewers, using 2 chicken pieces and 1 pineapple chunk per skewer.

3. Preheat grill. Grill skewers 6" from medium coals for 8–12 minutes, turning frequently, until chicken is cooked. Sprinkle with lime juice and serve immediately.

CALORIES: 119.37 | Fat: 3.54g | Saturated fat: 1.33g | Dietary fiber: 0.44g | Sodium: 40.24mg | Cholesterol: 45.18mg

High-Fiber Guacamole

Lima beans and peas add fiber to this delicious low-fat guacamole. Remember that avocados have lots of heart-healthy monounsaturated fat and are low in saturated fat.

INGREDIENTS | YIELDS 3 CUPS; SERVING SIZE ¼ CUP

1 tablespoon olive oil

1 onion, finely chopped

3 cloves garlic, minced

1 10-ounce package frozen baby lima beans

1 cup frozen peas

2 avocados

2 tablespoons lemon juice

¼ teaspoon salt

½ cup low-fat sour cream

½ teaspoon crushed red pepper flakes

1. In medium saucepan, heat olive oil over medium heat. Add onion and garlic; cook and stir until crisp-tender. Add lima beans; cook and stir for 3 minutes, then add peas; cook and stir for 2–4 minutes longer until peas and lima beans are tender. Remove from heat and cool for 20 minutes.

2. Peel avocado, cut in half, remove pit, and place in medium bowl and top with lemon juice and salt. Add lima bean/pea mixture, and mash. Blend in sour cream and red pepper flakes. Serve immediately, or cover and refrigerate up to 4 hours before serving.

CALORIES: 129.39 | Fat: 7.59g | Saturated fat: 1.94g | Dietary fiber: 4.88g | Sodium: 79.72mg | Cholesterol: 3.93mg

Greek Quesadillas

Quesadillas can be made with any ethnic ingredients. Try sun-dried tomatoes, basil, and Parmesan cheese for Italian quesadillas.

INGREDIENTS | SERVES 8

1 cucumber

1 cup plain yogurt

½ teaspoon dried oregano leaves

1 tablespoon lemon juice

½ cup crumbled feta cheese

4 green onions, chopped

3 plum tomatoes, chopped

1 cup fresh baby spinach leaves

1 cup shredded part-skim mozzarella cheese

12 6" no-salt corn tortillas

1. Peel cucumber, remove seeds, and chop. In small bowl, combine cucumber with yogurt, oregano, and lemon juice and set aside.

2. In medium bowl, combine feta cheese, green onions, tomatoes, baby spinach, and mozzarella cheese and mix well.

3. Preheat griddle or skillet. Place six tortillas on work surface. Divide tomato mixture among them. Top with remaining tortillas and press down gently.

4. Cook quesadillas, pressing down occasionally with spatula, until tortillas are lightly browned. Flip quesadillas and cook on second side until tortillas are crisp and cheese is melted. Cut quesadillas in quarters and serve with yogurt mixture.

CALORIES: 84.35 | Fat: 6.03g | Saturated fat: 1.31g | Dietary fiber: 0.06g | Sodium: 44.06mg | Cholesterol: 3.67mg

Tortillas

Tortillas are made with flour or with corn. They may have no fat, but the typical 10" flour tortilla made with salt has about 400mg of sodium! Read labels carefully to find no-salt tortillas. Flour tortillas are flavored with everything from spinach to red peppers to tomatoes. Corn tortillas have more nutrition and more fiber.

Yogurt Cheese Balls

Make sure the yogurt you use to make yogurt cheese is free of fillers and thickening agents; find the purest yogurt possible.

INGREDIENTS | SERVES 8

2 cups plain low-fat yogurt

¼ cup minced flat-leaf parsley

¼ cup minced chives

3 tablespoons extra-virgin olive oil

1 tablespoon aged balsamic vinegar

Yogurt Cheese

Use yogurt cheese as a substitute for sour cream in most recipes. Mix it with some herbs and spices and use it to top a baked potato. And it's a perfect appetizer dip combined with everything from salsa to pesto.

1. To make the yogurt cheese, the day before, line a strainer with cheesecloth. Place the strainer in a large bowl and add the yogurt. Cover and refrigerate overnight. The next day, place the thickened yogurt in a medium bowl. Discard the liquid, or whey, or reserve for use in soups and gravies.

2. Roll the yogurt cheese into 1" balls. On shallow plate, combine parsley and chives. Roll yogurt balls in herbs to coat. Place on serving plate and drizzle with olive oil and vinegar. Serve immediately.

CALORIES: 181.26 | Fat: 6.34g | Saturated fat: 3.62g | Dietary fiber: 2.75g | Sodium: 208.14mg | Cholesterol: 17.67mg

Creamy Garlic Hummus

Hummus, made from garbanzo beans, is an excellent source of folate and soluble fiber. Plus, it tastes great!

INGREDIENTS | SERVES 6–8

1 head roasted garlic

1 15-ounce can no-salt garbanzo beans

½ cup Yogurt Cheese (as described in recipe for Yogurt Cheese Balls, see previous recipe)

2 tablespoons lemon juice

¼ cup tahini

2 tablespoons olive oil

3 tablespoons toasted sesame seeds

1. Remove roasted garlic from the papery skins and place in blender or food processor. Rinse and drain garbanzo beans and add to blender along with Yogurt Cheese, lemon juice, and tahini.

2. Blend or process until smooth. Place in serving bowl and drizzle with olive oil. Sprinkle with sesame seeds and serve with breadsticks, pita chips, and crackers.

CALORIES: 231.54 | Fat: 11.71g | Saturated fat: 1.57g | Dietary fiber: 5.41g | Sodium: 26.76mg | Cholesterol: 16.78mg

Corn Polenta Chowder

*Turkey bacon helps reduce the fat in this excellent thick chowder,
but it is high in salt, so no additional salt is needed.*

INGREDIENTS | SERVES 6

2 strips turkey bacon

1 tablespoon olive oil

1 red onion, chopped

3 cloves garlic, minced

1 red bell pepper, chopped

2 jalapeño peppers, minced

2 Yukon Gold potatoes, chopped

5 cups Low-Sodium Chicken Broth (see recipe in this chapter)

⅓ cup cornmeal

2 tablespoons adobo sauce

2 10-ounce packages frozen corn, thawed

1 cup fat-free half-and-half

¼ cup chopped cilantro

⅛ teaspoon cayenne pepper

1. In a large soup pot, cook bacon until crisp. Remove from heat, crumble, and set aside. To drippings remaining in pot, add olive oil, then onion and garlic; cook and stir until tender, about 5 minutes.

2. Stir in bell pepper, jalapeños, potatoes, and 3 cups of the broth. Bring to a boil, then reduce heat, cover, and simmer for 20 minutes until potatoes are tender.

3. Meanwhile, in a small microwave-safe bowl, combine cornmeal and 1 cup chicken broth. Microwave on high for 2 minutes, remove and stir, then microwave for 2–4 minutes longer or until mixture thickens; stir in adobo sauce and remaining 1 cup chicken broth. Add to soup along with corn. Simmer for another 10 minutes.

4. Add the half-and-half, cilantro, and cayenne pepper and stir well. Heat until steam rises, then sprinkle with reserved bacon and serve immediately.

CALORIES: 276.10 | Fat: 6.03g | Saturated fat: 1.42g | Dietary fiber: 5.22g | Sodium: 184.32mg | Cholesterol: 6.22mg

Red Lentil Soup

This is a great, hearty soup that freezes well. Make an extra batch and freeze it for those days when you don't feel like cooking.

INGREDIENTS	SERVES 4

2 tablespoons olive oil

4 cloves garlic, minced

1 cup chopped onion

2 tablespoons minced gingerroot

2 parsnips, peeled and chopped

3 carrots, peeled and chopped

2 cups vegetable broth

2 cups water

2 sprigs fresh thyme

1 cup red lentils

1. In a large soup pot, heat olive oil over medium heat. Add garlic and onion; cook and stir until crisp-tender, about 4 minutes. Add gingerroot, parsnips, and carrots and cook for 2 minutes. Then stir in vegetable broth, water, and thyme sprigs and bring to a boil. Reduce heat, cover, and simmer for 10 minutes.

2. Meanwhile, pick over lentils and wash thoroughly. Add lentils to pot and bring back to a simmer. Simmer for 15–25 minutes or until lentils and vegetables are tender. Remove the thyme stems and discard. You can purée this soup if you'd like, but you can also serve just as it is.

CALORIES: 271.98 | Fat: 8.05g | Saturated fat: 1.24g | Dietary fiber: 15.32g | Sodium: 41.12mg | Cholesterol: 0.0mg

Beans for Soup

Since beans and legumes are so full of fiber and a great way to reduce cholesterol, you should eat lots of them. Unfortunately, canned beans are very high in sodium. Make up a batch of these beans and freeze them, then use instead of canned beans.

INGREDIENTS	YIELDS 10 CUPS; SERVING SIZE 1 CUP

1 pound dried beans

Water, as needed

Ready to Use

To use, defrost in refrigerator overnight, or open bag and microwave on defrost until beans begin thawing, then stir into soup to heat.

1. Sort beans, then rinse well and drain. Combine in a large pot with water to cover by 1". Bring to a boil, cover pan, remove from heat, and let stand for 2 hours.

2. Refrigerate pot and let beans soak overnight. In the morning, drain and rinse; drain again. Place in a 5- to 6-quart slow cooker with water to just cover. Cover and cook on low for 8–10 hours until beans are tender.

3. Package beans in 1-cup portions into freezer bags, including a bit of the cooking liquid. Freeze for up to 3 months.

CALORIES: 219.48 | Fat: 0.16g | Saturated fat: 0.03g | Dietary fiber: 16.46g | Sodium: 7.08mg | Cholesterol: 0.0mg

Scandinavian Summer Fruit Soup

This is wonderful for a summer brunch. To make this a winter soup, use dried fruits like raisins and apricots. Each serving of soup gives you more than 100 percent of your daily requirement of vitamin C.

INGREDIENTS | SERVES 6

4 cups apple cider

1 cup cranberry juice

½ cup orange juice

¼ cup lemon juice

¼ cup sugar

¼ teaspoon salt

4 peaches, peeled and chopped

1 pint strawberries, chopped

2 pears, peeled and chopped

2 cinnamon sticks

½ teaspoon ground cardamom

1 bunch fresh mint

6 tablespoons low-fat sour cream

1. Make the soup the day before. In a large bowl, combine apple cider, cranberry juice, orange juice, lemon juice, sugar, and salt.

2. Place half of the peaches, strawberries, and pears in a food processor or blender. Add 1 cup of the apple cider mixture and blend or process until smooth. Add to apple cider mixture along with remaining ingredients except mint and sour cream. Cover and chill for at least 8 hours.

3. Remove cinnamon sticks and stir soup. Then spoon soup into chilled bowls and garnish with mint and sour cream.

CALORIES: 241.46 | Fat: 2.49g | Saturated fat: 1.19g | Dietary fiber: 4.13g | Sodium: 111.65mg | Cholesterol: 5.85mg

Fresh Yellow Tomato Soup

This light soup is a fine starter for a formal dinner party or for a late-summer lunch when tomatoes, basil, and peppers are at their peak.

INGREDIENTS | SERVES 6

Water, as needed

8 yellow tomatoes

1 tablespoon olive oil

1 tablespoon butter

4 cloves garlic, peeled and minced

1 yellow bell pepper, chopped

1 red bell pepper, chopped

4 cups Low-Sodium Chicken Broth (see recipe in this chapter)

1 tablespoon lemon juice

⅛ teaspoon white pepper

1 large bunch basil, torn

¼ cup toasted sliced almonds

1. Prepare a large bowl of ice water. Bring large pot of water to a boil. Cut an X into the bottom of each tomato and drop tomatoes into boiling water. Bring water back to a boil and simmer for 1 minute, then remove each tomato and drop into ice water. Let cool for 5 minutes, then peel tomatoes; discard skin.

2. Heat a large soup pot over medium heat and add olive oil and butter and let melt. Add garlic; cook and stir for 3 minutes. Cut tomatoes into quarters and add to pot along with peppers. Cook and stir for 4 minutes.

3. Add the broth, lemon juice, and pepper. Bring to a boil and cook for 10 minutes, then add half of the basil.

4. Using an immersion blender, purée soup. Or purée soup in batches in a blender or food processor. Garnish with remaining basil and toasted almonds and serve.

CALORIES: 197.11 | Fat: 11.57g | Saturated fat: 3.08g | Dietary fiber: 3.99g | Sodium: 158.84mg | Cholesterol: 7.63mg

Low-Sodium Beef Broth

Even low-sodium varieties of canned beef broth have large amounts of sodium, about 400mg per cup. This rich broth has hardly any sodium, but it does have lots of flavor.

INGREDIENTS | YIELDS 10 CUPS

3 pounds soup bones

1 pound beef shank

4 carrots, cut into 1" chunks

2 onions, chopped

2 tablespoons olive oil

2 bay leaves

5 cloves garlic, crushed

5 peppercorns

8 cups water

Making Broth

The secrets to making a rich broth include thoroughly browning the bones and vegetables and also letting the broth simmer a long time. You can also clarify the broth; after the fat is removed, bring the broth to a boil with the shell of an egg. Simmer for 5 minutes, then strain the broth through several layers of cheesecloth or a coffee strainer.

1. Preheat oven to 400°F. In a large roasting pan, place soup bones, beef shank, carrots, and onions. Drizzle with olive oil and toss to coat. Roast for 2 hours or until bones and vegetables are brown.

2. Place roasted bones and vegetables along with bay leaves, garlic, and peppercorns in a 5- to 6-quart slow cooker. Pour 1 cup water into roasting pan and scrape up brown bits; add to slow cooker. Then pour remaining water into slow cooker. Cover and cook on low for 8–9 hours.

3. Strain broth into a large bowl; discard solids. Cover broth and refrigerate overnight. In the morning, remove fat solidified on surface and discard. Pour broth into freezer containers. Seal, label, and freeze up to 3 months. To use, defrost in refrigerator overnight.

CALORIES: 31.45 | Fat: 0.88g | Saturated fat: 0.29g | Dietary fiber: 0.11g | Sodium: 15.65mg | Cholesterol: 8.85mg

Low-Sodium Chicken Broth

Browning the chicken before making stock adds rich flavor and deepens the color.

INGREDIENTS | YIELDS 8 CUPS; SERVING SIZE 1 CUP

2 tablespoons olive oil
3 pounds cut-up chicken
2 onions, chopped
5 cloves garlic, minced
4 carrots, sliced
4 stalks celery, sliced
1 tablespoon peppercorns
1 bay leaf
6 cups water
2 tablespoons lemon juice

1. In a large skillet, heat olive oil over medium heat. Add chicken, skin-side down, and cook until browned, about 8–10 minutes. Place chicken in a 5- to 6-quart slow cooker.

2. Add onions and garlic to drippings in skillet; cook and stir for 2–3 minutes, scraping bottom of skillet. Add to slow cooker along with remaining ingredients except lemon juice. Cover and cook on low for 8–9 hours.

3. Strain broth into a large bowl. Remove meat from chicken; refrigerate or freeze for another use. Cover broth and refrigerate overnight. In the morning, remove fat solidified on surface and discard. Stir in lemon juice.

CALORIES: 82.89 | Fat: 5.22g | Saturated fat: 0.92mg | Dietary fiber: 0.66g | Sodium: 39.09mg | Cholesterol: 17.86mg

Crisp Polenta with Tomato Sauce

Crisp and crunchy polenta is served with hot pasta sauce in this simple recipe.

INGREDIENTS | SERVES 8

1 recipe Cheese Polenta (see recipe in this chapter)
1 cup shredded part-skim mozzarella cheese
3 cups Spaghetti Sauce (Chapter 18), heated

1. Prepare polenta as directed. When done, pour onto a greased cookie sheet; spread to a ½"-thick rectangle, about 9" × 15". Cover and chill until very firm, about 2 hours.

2. Preheat broiler. Cut polenta into fifteen 3" squares. Place on a broiler pan; broil for 4–6 minutes or until golden-brown. Carefully turn polenta and broil until golden-brown.

3. Remove from oven and sprinkle with mozzarella cheese. Top each with a dollop of the hot Spaghetti Sauce, and serve immediately.

CALORIES: 229.70 | Fat: 8.43g | Saturated fat: 4.20g | Dietary fiber: 3.46g | Sodium: 260.08mg | Cholesterol: 17.91mg

Vegetable-Barley Stew

This amount of meat adds rich flavor without increasing the cholesterol or saturated-fat content of the stew.

INGREDIENTS | SERVES 8

¾ pound beef round steak

2 tablespoons flour

1 teaspoon paprika

2 tablespoons olive oil

2 onions, chopped

4 cups Low-Sodium Beef Broth (see recipe in this chapter), divided

4 carrots, thickly sliced

3 potatoes, cubed

1 8-ounce package sliced mushrooms

3 cups water

1 teaspoon dried marjoram leaves

1 bay leaf

¼ teaspoon salt

¼ teaspoon pepper

¾ cup hulled barley

1. Trim beef and cut into 1" pieces. Sprinkle with flour and paprika and toss to coat. In a large skillet, heat olive oil over medium heat. Add beef; brown beef, stirring occasionally, for about 5–6 minutes. Remove to a 4- to 5-quart slow cooker.

2. Add onions to skillet along with ½ cup beef broth. Bring to a boil, then simmer, scraping the bottom of the skillet, for 3–4 minutes. Add to slow cooker along with all remaining ingredients.

3. Cover and cook on low for 8–9 hours, or until barley and vegetables are tender. Stir, remove bay leaf, and serve immediately.

CALORIES: 295.45 | Fat: 9.45g | Saturated fat: 2.59g | Dietary fiber: 6.02g | Sodium: 250.21mg | Cholesterol: 42.67mg

Barley

Barley contains a substance called beta-glucan that has proved effective in reducing cholesterol levels in clinical studies. You can buy barley in several forms. Hulled barley is the most nutritious, while pearl barley is more polished and cooks more quickly. Barley flakes and grits are also available for quick-cooking recipes.

Three Bean Chili

*Chili without meat but with beans is rich and satisfying. If you love hot food,
use habanero peppers instead of the jalapeños.*

INGREDIENTS | SERVES 6

1 cup dried black beans

1 cup dried kidney beans

1 cup dried pinto beans

Water, as needed, plus 4 cups

2 jalapeño peppers, minced

2 onions, chopped

4 cloves garlic, minced

4 cups Low-Sodium Beef Broth (see
recipe in this chapter), divided

2 14-ounce cans low-sodium diced
tomatoes, undrained

1 6-ounce can low-sodium tomato paste

⅛ teaspoon pepper

1. Pick over beans and rinse well; drain and place in large bowl. Cover with water and let stand overnight. In the morning, drain and rinse the beans and place them into a 4- to 5-quart slow cooker.

2. Add peppers, onions, and garlic to slow cooker. Add 4 cups water and 3 cups broth to the slow cooker. Stir well. Cover and cook on low for 8 hours, or until beans are tender.

3. Add canned tomatoes to slow cooker. In a small bowl, combine remaining 1 cup broth with the tomato paste; stir with whisk to dissolve the tomato paste. Add to slow cooker along with pepper. Cover and cook on low for 1–2 hours longer or until chili is thick.

CALORIES: 326.20 | Fat: 1.50g | Saturated fat: 0.36g | Dietary fiber: 16.52g | Sodium: 64.96mg | Cholesterol: 4.42mg

Potato Soufflé

This soufflé isn't as light as others; it's more like a potato puff. Serve it with a fruit salad for a nice lunch.

INGREDIENTS | SERVES 4

2 Yukon Gold potatoes
Water, as needed
1 tablespoon olive oil
⅛ teaspoon nutmeg
¼ teaspoon onion salt
⅛ teaspoon cayenne pepper
⅓ cup fat-free half-and-half
¼ cup grated Parmesan cheese
4 egg whites
¼ teaspoon cream of tartar
1 cup chopped grape tomatoes
¼ cup chopped fresh basil

Cooking Potatoes

When cooking with potatoes, place them in cold water to cover as you are peeling or chopping them. Potatoes can turn brown very quickly, and this slows the process. Do not overcook potatoes; cook them just until they are tender when pierced with a knife. Drain well and shake in the hot pot to remove excess moisture.

1. Preheat oven to 450°F. Peel and thinly slice potatoes, adding to a pot of cold water as you work. Bring potatoes to a boil over high heat, reduce heat, and simmer until tender, about 12–15 minutes.

2. Drain potatoes and return to hot pot; shake for 1 minute. Add olive oil, nutmeg, salt, and pepper and mash until smooth. Beat in the half-and-half and Parmesan.

3. In large bowl, combine egg whites with cream of tartar and beat until stiff peaks form. Stir a dollop of the egg whites into the potato mixture and stir. Then fold in remaining egg whites.

4. Spray the bottom of a 2-quart casserole dish with nonstick cooking spray. Spoon potato mixture into casserole. Bake for 20 minutes, then reduce heat to 375°F and bake for another 12–17 minutes or until soufflé is golden-brown and puffed.

5. While soufflé is baking, combine tomatoes and basil in small bowl and mix gently. Serve immediately with tomato mixture for topping the soufflé.

CALORIES: 224.39 | Fat: 9.11g | Saturated fat: 2.24g | Dietary fiber: 2.79g | Sodium: 260.97mg | Cholesterol: 6.51mg

Ratatouille

This rich vegetable stew can be served over brown rice, pasta, or couscous, either hot or cold.

INGREDIENTS | SERVES 6

3 tablespoons olive oil
2 onions, chopped
4 cloves garlic, minced
1 green bell pepper, sliced
1 yellow bell pepper, sliced
1 eggplant, peeled and cubed
¼ teaspoon salt
⅛ teaspoon pepper
2 tablespoons flour
2 zucchini, sliced
1 tablespoon red wine vinegar
2 tablespoons capers, rinsed
¼ cup chopped flat-leaf parsley

1. In a large saucepan, heat olive oil over medium heat. Add onion and garlic; cook and stir until crisp-tender, about 3 minutes. Add bell peppers; cook and stir until crisp-tender, about 3 minutes.

2. Sprinkle eggplant with salt, pepper, and flour. Add to saucepan; cook and stir until eggplant begins to soften. Add remaining ingredients except parsley; cover, and simmer for 30–35 minutes or until vegetables are soft and mixture is blended. Sprinkle with parsley and serve.

CALORIES: 124.26 | Fat: 7.10g | Saturated fat: 1.02g | Dietary fiber: 4.47g | Sodium: 187.22mg | Cholesterol: 0.0mg

Cheese Polenta

Polenta is a classic Italian dish that you can dress up many ways. Add fresh herbs, sautéed onion or other vegetables, or different cheeses to this basic recipe.

INGREDIENTS | SERVES 6

¼ teaspoon salt
3 cups water
1 cup skim milk
1¼ cups yellow cornmeal
1 tablespoon butter or plant sterol margarine
¼ cup grated Parmesan cheese
¼ cup shredded Havarti cheese
½ teaspoon crushed red pepper flakes

1. In large saucepan, combine salt and water and bring to a boil. In small bowl, combine milk with cornmeal and mix until smooth.

2. Slowly add the cornmeal mixture to the boiling water, stirring constantly with a wire whisk. Cook over medium-low heat, stirring constantly, until polenta is very thick, about 5–10 minutes. Stir in butter, cheeses, and red pepper flakes. Serve immediately.

CALORIES: 171.53 | Fat: 4.91g | Saturated fat: 2.85g | Dietary fiber: 2.13g | Sodium: 204.96mg | Cholesterol: 13.71mg

Chili Fries

You can double this recipe; bake it on two cookie sheets, rotating the sheets in the oven halfway through the cooking time.

INGREDIENTS | SERVES 4–6

4 russet potatoes
2 tablespoons olive oil
2 tablespoons chili powder
1 tablespoon grill seasoning
1 teaspoon ground cumin
1 teaspoon paprika
¼ teaspoon pepper

1. Preheat oven to 425°F. Scrub potatoes and pat dry; cut into ½" strips, leaving skin on. A few strips won't have any skin. Toss with olive oil and arrange in a single layer on a large cookie sheet.

2. In small bowl, combine remaining ingredients and mix well. Sprinkle over potatoes and toss to coat. Arrange in single layer.

3. Bake for 35–45 minutes, turning once during baking time, until potatoes are deep golden-brown and crisp.

CALORIES: 225.16 | Fat: 4.76g | Saturated fat: 0.69g | Dietary fiber: 4.39g | Sodium: 213.81mg | Cholesterol: 0.0mg

"Egg" Salad Sandwich Spread

Tofu's mild flavor can be seasoned many ways.
Use different spices and cheeses to vary this spread recipe.

INGREDIENTS | YIELDS 3 CUPS; SERVING SIZE ½ CUP

½ 12-ounce package firm tofu
⅓ cup low-fat mayonnaise
2 tablespoons plain yogurt
2 tablespoons Dijon mustard
⅛ teaspoon pepper
½ teaspoon dried oregano leaves
1 cup chopped celery
1 red bell pepper, chopped
¼ cup grated Parmesan cheese

1. Drain tofu and drain again on paper towels, pressing to remove moisture. Set aside.

2. In medium bowl, combine remaining ingredients and stir gently to combine. Crumble tofu into bowl and mix until mixture looks like egg salad. Cover tightly and refrigerate for 2–3 hours before serving. Store, covered, in the refrigerator for 3–4 days.

CALORIES: 105.78 | Fat: 7.17g | Saturated fat: 1.71g | Dietary fiber: 1.23g | Sodium: 235.50mg | Cholesterol: 3.97mg

Mini Hot-Pepper Pizzas

English-muffin pizzas are a classic snack. Using lots of peppers adds vitamin C, fiber, and great flavor.

INGREDIENTS | SERVES 4

4 whole-wheat English muffins, split

1 tablespoon olive oil

2 cloves garlic, minced

1 red bell pepper, diced

2 jalapeño peppers, minced

⅛ teaspoon pepper

½ teaspoon dried oregano leaves

½ cup part-skim ricotta cheese

¼ cup grated Parmesan cheese

English Muffins

English muffins are a great choice for sandwiches or a pizza base. Split the muffins with a fork to create peaks and ridges that hold ingredients and become crunchy when toasted or grilled. Whole-wheat or whole-grain English muffins are readily available. They do spoil rather quickly, so freeze them after the first day.

1. Preheat oven to broil. Place English muffins, split side up, on a broiler pan. Broil 6" from heat source until lightly toasted, about 3–5 minutes. Remove from oven and set aside.

2. In medium skillet, heat olive oil over medium heat. Add garlic, red pepper, and jalapeño. Cook and stir until tender, about 5 minutes. Sprinkle with pepper and oregano.

3. Stir ricotta into vegetable mixture; spread on the English muffin halves. Sprinkle with Parmesan. Broil 6" from heat source for 5–8 minutes or until pizzas are hot and topping bubbles and begins to brown. Let cool for 5 minutes, then serve.

CALORIES: 239.93 | Fat: 8.87g | Saturated fat: 3.26g | Dietary fiber: 3.57g | Sodium: 351.25mg | Cholesterol: 15.11mg

CHAPTER 17

Heart-Healthy Meat and Poultry Main-Dish Recipes

Sautéed Chicken with Roasted Garlic Sauce

When roasted, garlic turns sweet and nutty.
Combined with tender sautéed chicken, this makes a memorable meal.

INGREDIENTS | SERVES 4

1 head roasted garlic

⅓ cup Low-Sodium Chicken Broth (Chapter 16)

½ teaspoon dried oregano leaves

¼ cup flour

⅛ teaspoon salt

⅛ teaspoon pepper

¼ teaspoon paprika

4 4-ounce boneless, skinless chicken breasts

2 tablespoons olive oil

Chicken and Cholesterol

Chicken is fairly high in cholesterol, but it's very low in saturated fat. The American Heart Association has boneless, skinless chicken breasts on its approved foods list, so you don't have to worry. If you are susceptible to cholesterol in food, reduce the serving size to 3 ounces per person.

1. Squeeze garlic cloves from the skins and combine in small saucepan with chicken broth and oregano leaves.

2. On shallow plate, combine flour, salt, pepper, and paprika. Dip chicken into this mixture to coat.

3. In large skillet, heat 2 tablespoons olive oil. At the same time, place the saucepan with the garlic mixture over medium heat. Add the chicken to the hot olive oil; cook for 5 minutes without moving. Then carefully turn chicken and cook for 4–7 minutes longer until chicken is thoroughly cooked.

4. Stir garlic sauce with wire whisk until blended. Serve with the chicken.

CALORIES: 267.01 | Fat: 7.78g | Saturated fat: 1.65g | Dietary fiber: 0.69g | Sodium: 158.61mg | Cholesterol: 91.85mg

Asian Chicken Stir-Fry

Yellow summer squash is a thin-skinned squash like zucchini. It has a mild, sweet flavor.

INGREDIENTS | SERVES 4

2 5-ounce boneless, skinless chicken breasts

½ cup Low-Sodium Chicken Broth (Chapter 16)

1 tablespoon low-sodium soy sauce

1 tablespoon cornstarch

1 tablespoon sherry

2 tablespoons peanut oil

1 onion, sliced

3 cloves garlic, minced

1 tablespoon grated gingerroot

1 cup snow peas

½ cup canned sliced water chestnuts, drained

1 yellow summer squash, sliced

¼ cup chopped unsalted peanuts

1. Cut chicken into strips and set aside. In small bowl, combine chicken broth, soy sauce, cornstarch, and sherry and set aside.

2. In large skillet or wok, heat peanut oil over medium-high heat. Add chicken; stir-fry until almost cooked, about 3–4 minutes. Remove to plate. Add onion, garlic, and gingerroot to skillet; stir-fry for 4 minutes longer. Then add snow peas, water chestnuts, and squash; stir-fry for 2 minutes longer.

3. Stir chicken broth mixture and add to skillet along with chicken. Stir-fry for 3–4 minutes longer or until chicken is thoroughly cooked and sauce is thickened and bubbly. Sprinkle with peanuts and serve immediately.

CALORIES: 252.42 | Fat: 12.42g | Saturated fat: 2.06g | Dietary fiber: 3.36g | Sodium: 202.04mg | Cholesterol: 41.11mg

Chicken Spicy Thai-Style

Peanut butter thickens the sauce and adds rich flavor to this easy stir-fry without adding any cholesterol.

INGREDIENTS | SERVES 4

2 tablespoons lime juice

1 tablespoon low-sodium soy sauce

½ cup Low-Sodium Chicken Broth (Chapter 16)

¼ cup dry white wine

¼ cup natural peanut butter

2 tablespoons peanut oil

1 onion, chopped

4 cloves garlic, minced

3 4-ounce boneless, skinless chicken breasts, sliced

4 cups shredded Napa cabbage

1 cup shredded carrots

Natural Peanut Butter

Whenever possible, use natural peanut butter, not the regular kind found on store shelves. Read labels carefully. You'll notice that most regular peanut butter contains hydrogenated vegetable oil, which is a source of trans fat. The oil will separate out of the natural peanut butter as it stands; just stir it back in before using.

1. In a small bowl, combine lime juice, soy sauce, chicken broth, wine, and peanut butter and mix with wire whisk until blended. Set aside.

2. In a wok or large skillet, heat peanut oil over medium-high heat. Add onion and garlic; stir-fry until crisp-tender, about 4 minutes. Add chicken; stir-fry until almost cooked, about 3 minutes. Add cabbage and carrots; stir-fry until cabbage begins to wilt, about 3–4 minutes longer.

3. Remove food from wok and return wok to heat. Add peanut butter mixture and bring to a simmer. Return chicken and vegetables to wok; stir-fry until sauce bubbles and thickens and chicken is thoroughly cooked, about 3–4 minutes. Serve immediately.

CALORIES: 300.35 | Fat: 16.70g | Saturated fat: 3.20g | Dietary fiber: 2.16g | Sodium: 309.32mg | Cholesterol: 51.56mg

Chicken Breasts with New Potatoes

This easy one-dish meal has the best combination of flavors. Mustard adds a nice bit of spice to tender chicken and crisp potatoes.

INGREDIENTS | SERVES 6

12 small new red potatoes

2 tablespoons olive oil

⅛ teaspoon white pepper

4 cloves garlic, minced

1 teaspoon dried oregano leaves

2 tablespoons Dijon mustard

4 4-ounce boneless, skinless chicken breasts

1 cup cherry tomatoes

1. Preheat oven to 400°F. Line a roasting pan with parchment paper and set aside. Scrub potatoes and cut each in half. Place in prepared pan.

2. In a small bowl, combine oil, pepper, garlic, oregano, and mustard and mix well. Drizzle half of this mixture over the potatoes and toss to coat. Roast for 20 minutes.

3. Cut chicken breasts into quarters. Remove pan from oven and add chicken to potato mixture. Using a spatula, mix potatoes and chicken together. Drizzle with remaining oil mixture. Return to oven and roast for 15 minutes longer.

4. Add tomatoes to pan. Roast for 5–10 minutes longer, or until potatoes are tender and browned and chicken is thoroughly cooked.

CALORIES: 395.92 | Fat: 9.57g | Saturated fat: 1.85g | Dietary fiber: 5.21g | Sodium: 142.98mg | Cholesterol: 61.23mg

Hazelnut-Crusted Chicken Breasts

This super-quick dish is perfect for a last-minute dinner.
Serve with a spinach salad and some crisp breadsticks.

INGREDIENTS | SERVES 2

2 4-ounce boneless, skinless chicken
 breasts
Pinch salt
Pinch pepper
1 tablespoon Dijon mustard
1 egg white
⅓ cup chopped hazelnuts
1 tablespoon olive oil

1. Place chicken between two sheets of waxed paper. Pound, starting at center of chicken, until ¼" thick. Sprinkle chicken with salt and pepper. Spread each side of chicken with some of the mustard.

2. In small bowl, beat egg white until foamy. Dip chicken into egg white, then into hazelnuts, pressing to coat both sides.

3. In skillet, heat olive oil over medium heat. Add chicken; cook for 3 minutes without moving. Then carefully turn and cook for 1–3 minutes on second side until nuts are toasted.

CALORIES: 276.64 | Fat: 16.02g | Saturated fat: 1.88g | Dietary fiber: 1.46g | Sodium: 266.25mg | Cholesterol: 65.77mg

Hot-and-Spicy Peanut Thighs

Serve this easy and spicy recipe with whole-grain corn bread.

INGREDIENTS | SERVES 4

4 4-ounce chicken thighs
½ cup low-sodium barbecue sauce
2 teaspoons chili powder
½ cup chopped unsalted peanuts

Coating for Poultry

When you're baking poultry that has a nut or bread crumb coating, it's usually best to coat only the top side of the meat. The coating underneath can become mushy and fall off because of the moisture in the chicken. If you want to coat both sides, it's best to pan-fry or sauté the chicken, or bake it on a wire rack.

1. Preheat oven to 350°F. Spray a roasting pan with nonstick cooking spray and set aside. Pound chicken slightly, to ⅓" thickness.

2. In a shallow bowl, combine barbecue sauce and chili powder and mix well. Dip chicken into sauce, then dip one side into peanuts. Place, peanut side up, in prepared pan.

3. Bake for 30–40 minutes, or until chicken is thoroughly cooked and nuts are browned. Serve immediately.

CALORIES: 327.41 | Fat: 19.55g | Saturated fat: 4.22g | Dietary fiber: 2.08g | Sodium: 129.88mg | Cholesterol: 94.26mg

Sesame-Crusted Chicken

Nutty and crunchy sesame seeds make a delicious coating on tender chicken in this simple recipe.

INGREDIENTS | SERVES 4

2 tablespoons low-sodium soy sauce

2 cloves garlic, minced

1 tablespoon grated gingerroot

1 tablespoon brown sugar

1 teaspoon sesame oil

4 4-ounce boneless, skinless chicken breasts

½ cup sesame seeds

3 tablespoons olive oil

1 tablespoon butter

1. In a large, heavy-duty food-storage bag, combine soy sauce, garlic, gingerroot, brown sugar, and sesame oil and mix well. Add chicken; seal bag, and squish to coat chicken with marinade. Refrigerate for 8 hours.

2. When ready to eat, remove chicken from marinade; discard marinade. Dip chicken in sesame seeds to coat on all sides.

3. Heat olive oil and butter in large skillet over medium heat. Add chicken and cook for 5 minutes. Carefully turn chicken and cook for 3–6 minutes on second side.

CALORIES: 363.65 | Fat: 20.83g | Saturated fat: 4.15g | Dietary fiber: 2.24g | Sodium: 250.28mg | Cholesterol: 99.28mg

Turkey Breast with Dried Fruit

This is a good choice for smaller families celebrating Thanksgiving. The sauce is delicious over mashed potatoes or steamed brown rice.

INGREDIENTS | SERVES 6

1½ pounds bone-in turkey breast

⅛ teaspoon salt

⅛ teaspoon pepper

1 tablespoon flour

1 tablespoon olive oil

1 tablespoon butter

½ cup chopped prunes

½ cup chopped dried apricots

2 Granny Smith apples, peeled and chopped

1 cup Low-Sodium Chicken Broth (Chapter 16)

¼ cup Madeira wine

1. Sprinkle turkey with salt, pepper, and flour. In large saucepan, heat olive oil and butter over medium heat. Add turkey and cook until browned, about 5 minutes. Turn turkey.

2. Add all fruit to saucepan along with broth and wine. Cover and bring to a simmer. Reduce heat to medium-low and simmer for 55–65 minutes or until turkey is thoroughly cooked. Serve turkey with fruit and sauce.

CALORIES: 293.15 | Fat: 6.01g | Saturated fat: 1.94g | Dietary fiber: 1.89g | Sodium: 127.28mg | Cholesterol: 78.37mg

Texas BBQ Chicken Thighs

Make a double batch of this fabulous barbecue sauce all by itself in your slow cooker and freeze it in ¼-cup portions to use anytime.

INGREDIENTS | SERVES 6

2 tablespoons olive oil

1 onion, chopped

4 cloves garlic, minced

1 jalapeño pepper, minced

¼ cup orange juice

1 tablespoon low-sodium soy sauce

2 tablespoons apple-cider vinegar

2 tablespoons brown sugar

2 tablespoons Dijon mustard

1 14-ounce can crushed tomatoes, undrained

½ teaspoon cumin

1 tablespoon chili powder

¼ teaspoon pepper

6 4-ounce boneless, skinless chicken thighs

3 tablespoons cornstarch

¼ cup water

1. In a small skillet, heat olive oil over medium heat. Add onion and garlic; cook and stir until crisp-tender, about 4 minutes. Place in a 3-to-4 quart slow cooker and add jalapeño, orange juice, soy sauce, vinegar, brown sugar, mustard, tomatoes, cumin, chili powder, and pepper.

2. Add chicken to the sauce, pushing chicken into the sauce to completely cover. Cover and cook on low for 8–10 hours or until chicken is thoroughly cooked.

3. In a small bowl, combine cornstarch and water; stir until smooth. Add to slow cooker and stir. Cook on high for 15–20 minutes longer until sauce is thickened.

CALORIES: 236.53mg | Fat: 9.30g | Saturated fat: 1.79g | Dietary fiber: 1.76g | Sodium: 277.24mg | Cholesterol: 94.12mg

Chicken Thighs

Many people may consider chicken thighs too fatty. Though chicken thighs do contain more fat than skinless chicken breasts, they still have only 11g of fat per 4-ounce serving. That is less fat than one would find in the same-size serving of beef, lamb, or pork.

Turkey Cutlets Parmesan

This classic dish is usually smothered in cheese, with deep-fried breaded turkey.
This lighter version is just as delicious.

INGREDIENTS | SERVES 6

1 egg white

¼ cup dry bread crumbs

⅛ teaspoon pepper

4 tablespoons grated Parmesan cheese, divided

6 4-ounce turkey cutlets

2 tablespoons olive oil

1 15-ounce can no-salt tomato sauce

1 teaspoon dried Italian seasoning

½ cup finely shredded part-skim mozzarella cheese

1. Preheat oven to 350°F. Spray a 2-quart baking dish with nonstick cooking spray and set aside.

2. In a shallow bowl, beat egg white until foamy. On a plate, combine bread crumbs, pepper, and 2 tablespoons Parmesan. Dip the turkey cutlets into the egg white, then into the bread crumb mixture, turning to coat.

3. In a large saucepan, heat olive oil over medium heat. Add turkey cutlets; brown on both sides, about 2–3 minutes per side. Place in prepared baking dish. Add tomato sauce and Italian seasoning to a saucepan; bring to a boil.

4. Pour sauce over cutlets in baking pan and top with mozzarella cheese and remaining 2 tablespoons Parmesan. Bake for 25–35 minutes or until sauce bubbles and cheese melts and begins to brown. Serve with pasta, if desired.

CALORIES: 275.49 | Fat: 10.98g | Saturated fat: 3.43g | Dietary fiber: 1.55g | Sodium: 229.86mg | Cholesterol: 88.13mg

Turkey Curry with Fruit

This simple dish is fancy enough for company.
Serve it with brown-rice pilaf and some toasted whole-wheat French bread.

INGREDIENTS | SERVES 6

6 4-ounce turkey cutlets
1 tablespoon flour
1 tablespoon plus 1 teaspoon curry powder, divided
1 tablespoon olive oil
2 pears, chopped
1 apple, chopped
½ cup raisins
1 tablespoon sugar
⅛ teaspoon salt
⅓ cup apricot jam

1. Preheat oven to 350°F. Spray a cookie sheet with nonstick cooking spray. Arrange cutlets on cookie sheet. In small bowl, combine flour, 1 tablespoon curry powder, and olive oil and mix well. Spread evenly over cutlets.

2. In medium bowl, combine pears, apple, raisins, sugar, salt, 1 teaspoon curry powder, and apricot jam, and mix well. Divide this mixture over the turkey cutlets.

3. Bake for 35–45 minutes or until turkey is thoroughly cooked and fruit is hot and caramelized. Serve immediately.

CALORIES: 371.52 | Fat: 11.15g | Saturated fat: 2.80g | Dietary fiber: 3.22g | Sodium: 121.35mg | Cholesterol: 78.24mg

Chicken Pesto

Pesto can be made with any nut. Hazelnuts are especially good at lowering LDL cholesterol, and they're delicious in this green sauce.

INGREDIENTS | SERVES 6

1 cup packed fresh basil leaves
¼ cup toasted chopped hazelnuts
2 cloves garlic, chopped
2 tablespoons olive oil
1 tablespoon water
¼ cup grated Parmesan cheese
½ cup Low-Sodium Chicken Broth (Chapter 16)
12 ounces boneless, skinless chicken breasts
1 12-ounce package angel hair pasta

1. Bring a large pot of salted water to a boil. In a blender combine basil, hazelnuts, and garlic. Blend until very finely chopped. Add olive oil and water; blend until a paste forms. Then blend in Parmesan cheese; set aside.

2. In a large skillet, bring chicken broth to a simmer over medium heat. Cut chicken into strips and add to broth. Cook for 4 minutes, then add the pasta to the boiling water.

3. Cook pasta for 3–4 minutes, until al dente. Drain and add to chicken mixture; cook and stir until chicken is thoroughly cooked. Add basil mixture, remove from heat, and stir until a sauce forms. Serve immediately.

CALORIES: 373.68 | Fat: 11.06g | Saturated fat: 2.01g | Dietary fiber: 2.18g | Sodium: 108.92mg | Cholesterol: 38.04mg

Filet Mignon with Vegetables

This is a wonderful dish for entertaining. The roasted vegetables are tender and sweet, and the meat is juicy.

INGREDIENTS | SERVES 8–10

1 16-ounce package baby carrots, halved lengthwise

1 8-ounce package frozen pearl onions

16 new potatoes, halved

2 tablespoons olive oil

2 pounds filet mignon

⅛ teaspoon salt

⅛ teaspoon white pepper

½ cup dry red wine

1. Preheat oven to 425°F. Place carrots, onions, and potatoes in a large roasting pan and drizzle with olive oil; toss to coat. Spread in an even layer. Roast for 15 minutes, then remove from oven.

2. Top with filet mignon; sprinkle the meat with salt and pepper. Pour wine over meat and vegetables.

3. Return to oven; roast for 20–30 minutes longer until beef registers 150°F for medium. Remove from oven, tent with foil, and let stand for 5 minutes, then carve to serve.

CALORIES: 442.64 | Fat: 11.83g | Saturated fat: 3.77g | Dietary fiber: 6.06g | Sodium: 140.70mg | Cholesterol: 70.55mg

Beef with Mushroom Kabobs

Serve these kabobs with cooked brown rice, a tomato and spinach salad, and Silken Chocolate Mousse (Chapter 19) for dessert.

INGREDIENTS | SERVES 4

¼ cup dry red wine

1 tablespoon olive oil

⅛ teaspoon salt

⅛ teaspoon cayenne pepper

1 tablespoon dried basil leaves

2 cloves garlic, minced

1 pound beef sirloin steak

½ pound button mushrooms

½ pound cremini mushrooms

1 tablespoon lemon juice

1. In a medium glass bowl, combine wine, olive oil, salt, pepper, basil leaves, and garlic, and mix well. Cut steak into 1½" cubes and add to wine mixture. Stir to coat, cover, and refrigerate for 1 hour.

2. Preheat grill. Drain steak, reserving marinade. Trim mushroom stems and discard; brush mushrooms with lemon juice. Thread steak and mushrooms onto skewers.

3. Grill for 7–10 minutes, turning once and brushing with marinade, until beef is deep golden-brown and mushrooms are tender. Discard remaining marinade.

CALORIES: 215.70 | Fat: 7.08g | Saturated fat: 2.39g | Dietary fiber: 1.42g | Sodium: 101.33mg | Cholesterol: 78.63mg

Sirloin Meatballs in Sauce

Cooking meatballs in a sauce keeps them moist and tender.
Serve this with hot cooked pasta or brown rice.

**INGREDIENTS | SERVES 6; SERVING SIZE
2 MEATBALLS**

1 tablespoon olive oil

3 cloves garlic, minced

½ cup minced onion

2 egg whites

½ cup dry bread crumbs

¼ cup grated Parmesan cheese

½ teaspoon crushed fennel seeds

½ teaspoon dried oregano leaves

2 teaspoons Worcestershire sauce

⅛ teaspoon pepper

⅛ teaspoon crushed red pepper flakes

1 pound 95 percent lean ground sirloin

1 recipe Spaghetti Sauce (Chapter 18)

1. In a small saucepan, heat olive oil over medium heat. Add garlic and onion; cook and stir until tender, about 5 minutes. Remove from heat and place in a large mixing bowl.

2. Add egg whites, bread crumbs, Parmesan, fennel, oregano, Worcestershire sauce, pepper, and pepper flakes and mix well. Add sirloin; mix gently but thoroughly until combined. Form into 12 meatballs.

3. In large nonstick saucepan, place Spaghetti Sauce and bring to a simmer. Carefully add meatballs to sauce. Return to a simmer, partially cover, and simmer for 15–25 minutes or until meatballs are thoroughly cooked.

CALORIES: 367.93 | Fat: 13.56g | Saturated fat: 3.91g | Dietary fiber: 5.58g | Sodium: 305.47mg | Cholesterol: 61.12mg

Baking Meatballs

You can also bake these meatballs and freeze them plain to use in other recipes like Meatball Pizza (see recipe in this chapter). Place meatballs on a cookie sheet. Bake at 375°F for 15–25 minutes or until meatballs are browned and cooked through. Cool for 30 minutes, then chill until cold. Freeze individually in freezer bags. To thaw, let stand in refrigerator overnight.

Steak with Mushroom Sauce

A rich mushroom sauce adds great flavor to tender marinated steak. This is a recipe for company!

INGREDIENTS | **SERVES 6**

1 to 1¼ pounds flank steak

2 tablespoons red wine

1 tablespoon olive oil

1 tablespoon butter

1 onion, minced

1 8-ounce package sliced mushrooms

2 tablespoons flour

1½ cups Low-Sodium Beef Broth (Chapter 16)

¼ teaspoon ground coriander

2 teaspoons Worcestershire sauce

⅛ teaspoon pepper

1. In a glass dish, combine flank steak, red wine, and olive oil. Cover and marinate for at least 8 hours.

2. When ready to eat, prepare and preheat grill. Drain steak, reserving marinade.

3. In a large skillet, melt butter over medium heat. Add onion and mushrooms; cook and stir until liquid evaporates, about 8–9 minutes. Stir in flour; cook and stir for 2 minutes. Add beef broth and marinade from beef and bring to a boil. Stir in coriander, Worcestershire sauce, and pepper; reduce heat to low and simmer while cooking steak.

4. Cook steak 6" from medium coals for 7–10 minutes, turning once, until steak reaches desired doneness. Remove from heat, cover, and let stand for 10 minutes. Slice thinly against the grain and serve with mushroom sauce.

CALORIES: 262.45 | Fat: 16.09g | Saturated fat: 6.42g | Dietary fiber: 0.72g | Sodium: 114.22mg | Cholesterol: 53.86mg

Asian Beef Kabobs

Make sure that the wasabi powder is completely mixed with the olive oil before proceeding with the recipe, so the strong taste is evenly distributed.

INGREDIENTS | SERVES 4

2 tablespoons olive oil
1 teaspoon wasabi powder
1 tablespoon low-sodium soy sauce
1 tablespoon lemon juice
2 red bell peppers, sliced
1 8-ounce package cremini mushrooms
1 zucchini, sliced ½" thick
1 pound beef sirloin steak, cubed

1. In a small bowl, combine olive oil and wasabi powder; mix well. Add soy sauce and lemon juice and mix well.

2. Thread vegetables and steak on skewers. Brush with the marinade and let stand for 10 minutes.

3. Preheat grill. Grill skewers 6" from medium coals for 7–10 minutes, turning once and brushing with wasabi mixture several times, until beef reaches desired doneness and vegetables are crisp-tender. Serve immediately.

CALORIES: 254.80 | Fat: 9.55g | Saturated fat: 2.76g | Dietary fiber: 3.43g | Sodium: 217.78mg | Cholesterol: 81.36mg

Steak-and-Pepper Kabobs

Serve these kabobs with a rice pilaf and a mixed fruit salad.

INGREDIENTS | SERVES 4

2 tablespoons brown sugar
½ teaspoon garlic powder
⅛ teaspoon cayenne pepper
¼ teaspoon onion salt
½ teaspoon chili powder
⅛ teaspoon ground cloves
1 1-pound sirloin steak, cut in 1" cubes
2 red bell peppers, cut in strips
2 green bell peppers, cut in strips

1. In a small bowl, combine brown sugar, garlic powder, cayenne pepper, onion salt, chili powder, and cloves, and mix well. Toss sirloin steak with brown sugar mixture. Place in a glass dish and cover; refrigerate for 2 hours.

2. When ready to cook, prepare and preheat grill. Thread steak cubes and pepper strips on metal skewers. Grill 6" from medium coals for 5–8 minutes, turning once, until steak reaches desired doneness and peppers are crisp-tender. Serve immediately.

CALORIES: 205.53 | Fat: 6.23g | Saturated fat: 2.24g | Dietary fiber: 3.03g | Sodium: 133.03mg | Cholesterol: 58.54mg

Whole-Grain Meatloaf

For a delicious lunch, save some of this meatloaf to use in meatloaf sandwiches.

INGREDIENTS | SERVES 8

1 tablespoon olive oil

1 onion, finely chopped

3 cloves garlic, minced

1 cup minced mushrooms

⅛ teaspoon pepper

1 teaspoon dried marjoram leaves

1 egg

1 egg white

½ cup chili sauce

¼ cup milk

1 tablespoon Worcestershire sauce

4 slices whole-grain oatmeal bread

8 ounces 85 percent lean ground beef

8 ounces ground turkey

8 ounces ground pork

3 tablespoons ketchup

Meatloaf Secrets

There are a few tricks to making the best meatloaf. First, combine all the other ingredients and mix well, then add the meat last. The less the meat is handled, the more tender the meatloaf will be. Then, when it's done baking, remove from the oven, cover with foil, and let sit for 10 minutes to let the juices redistribute.

1. Preheat oven to 325°F. Spray a 9" × 5" loaf pan with nonstick cooking spray and set aside. In a large saucepan, heat olive oil over medium heat. Add onion, garlic, and mushrooms; cook and stir until tender, about 6 minutes. Place in large mixing bowl, sprinkle with pepper and marjoram, and let stand for 15 minutes.

2. Add egg, egg white, chili sauce, milk, and Worcestershire sauce, and mix well. Make crumbs from the oatmeal bread and add to onion mixture.

3. Add all of the meat and work gently with your hands just until combined. Press into prepared loaf pan. Top with ketchup. Bake for 60–75 minutes, or until internal temperature registers 165°F. Remove from oven, cover with foil, and let stand for 10 minutes before slicing.

CALORIES: 325.29 | Fat: 15.51g | Saturated fat: 4.70g | Dietary fiber: 2.18g | Sodium: 184.45mg | Cholesterol: 90.46mg

Corned Beef Hash

Serve this delicious hash on toasted Three-Grain French Bread (Chapter 19),
topped with scrambled eggs made with egg substitute.

INGREDIENTS | SERVES 6

2 tablespoons olive oil

2 onions, chopped

4 cloves garlic, minced

8 fingerling potatoes, chopped

4 carrots, chopped

¼ cup water

½ pound deli corned beef, diced

⅛ teaspoon ground cloves

⅛ teaspoon white pepper

3 tablespoons low-sodium chili sauce

1. Place olive oil in a large saucepan; heat over medium heat. Add onion and garlic; cook and stir for 3 minutes. Add potatoes and carrots; cook and stir until potatoes are partially cooked, about 5 minutes.

2. Add water, corned beef, cloves, pepper, and chili sauce. Stir well, then cover, reduce heat to low, and simmer for 10–15 minutes or until blended and potatoes are cooked. Serve immediately.

CALORIES: 283.21 | Fat: 11.97g | Saturated fat: 3.09g | Dietary fiber: 4.88g | Sodium: 472.63mg | Cholesterol: 37.02mg

Stuffed Meatloaf

A savory mushroom and bread filling adds great flavor and texture to this hearty meatloaf.

INGREDIENTS | SERVES 8

1 tablespoon butter

1 onion, chopped

1 8-ounce package sliced mushrooms

½ 10-ounce package frozen spinach, thawed and drained

1 recipe Whole-Grain Meatloaf (see recipe in this chapter), uncooked

2 tablespoons ketchup

2 tablespoons mustard

1. Preheat oven to 350°F. Spray a 9" × 5" loaf pan with nonstick cooking spray and set aside. In medium saucepan, melt butter over medium heat. Add onion and mushrooms; cook and stir for 3 minutes. Add spinach; cook until the vegetables are tender and the liquid evaporates.

2. Press half of the meatloaf mixture into prepared pan. Top with mushroom mixture, keeping away from sides of pan. Top with remaining meatloaf mixture.

3. In bowl, mix ketchup and mustard. Spoon over meatloaf. Bake for 55–65 minutes or until internal temperature registers 165°F. Cut into slices and serve.

CALORIES: 362.10 | Fat: 17.28g | Saturated fat: 5.65g | Dietary fiber: 3.44g | Sodium: 258.17mg | Cholesterol: 94.27mg

Meatball Pizza

Your own homemade pizza is always going to taste better than delivery!

INGREDIENTS | SERVES 6

1 tablespoon olive oil

1 onion, chopped

1 green bell pepper, chopped

½ cup shredded carrots

1 6-ounce can no-salt tomato paste

2 tablespoons mustard

¼ cup water

1 whole-grain pizza crust, prebaked

12 plain Sirloin Meatballs (see recipe in this chapter), baked

1 cup shredded extra-sharp Cheddar cheese

½ cup shredded part-skim mozzarella cheese

1. Preheat oven to 400°F. In a saucepan, heat olive oil over medium heat. Add onion, bell pepper, and carrots; cook and stir until crisp-tender. Add tomato paste, mustard, and water and bring to a simmer. Simmer, stirring frequently, for 5 minutes.

2. Spread the sauce over the pizza crust. Cut the meatballs in half and arrange on the pizza. Sprinkle with Cheddar and mozzarella cheeses.

3. Bake for 20–30 minutes. Let stand for 5 minutes, then serve.

CALORIES: 437.80 | Fat: 15.85g | Saturated fat: 6.29g | Dietary fiber: 4.88g | Sodium: 432.76mg | Cholesterol: 61.04mg

Whole-Wheat Spaghetti and Meatballs

This simple recipe is full of vitamins C and A. Serve it with toasted Three-Grain French Bread (Chapter 19) and some red wine.

INGREDIENTS | SERVES 6–8

1 recipe Sirloin Meatballs in Sauce (see recipe in this chapter)

1 8-ounce can no-salt tomato sauce

½ cup grated carrots

1 16-ounce package whole-wheat spaghetti

½ cup grated Parmesan cheese, divided

1. Bring a large pot of water to boil. Prepare the Sirloin Meatballs in Sauce, adding tomato sauce and grated carrots to the sauce. Simmer until meatballs are cooked.

2. Cook spaghetti in water according to package directions. Drain, reserving ¼ cup cooking water. Add spaghetti to meatballs in sauce along with ¼ cup of the cheese. Simmer, stirring gently, for 5–6 minutes, adding reserved cooking water if necessary for desired sauce consistency. Sprinkle with the remaining ¼ cup Parmesan cheese and serve immediately.

CALORIES: 386.78 | Fat: 12.34g | Saturated fat: 4.08g | Dietary fiber: 7.47g | Sodium: 444.23mg | Cholesterol: 51.34mg

Beef Risotto

This elegant recipe is perfect for a spring dinner.
It is a last-minute recipe, so don't start it until after your guests have arrived.

INGREDIENTS | SERVES 6

2 cups water

2 cups Low-Sodium Beef Broth (Chapter 16)

2 tablespoons olive oil

½ pound sirloin steak, chopped

1 onion, minced

2 cloves garlic, minced

1½ cups Arborio rice

2 tablespoons steak sauce

¼ teaspoon pepper

1 pound asparagus, cut into 2" pieces

¼ cup grated Parmesan cheese

1 tablespoon butter

1. In a medium saucepan, combine water and broth; heat over low heat until warm; keep on heat.

2. In a large saucepan, heat olive oil over medium heat. Add beef; cook and stir until browned. Remove from pan with slotted spoon and set aside. Add onion and garlic to pan; cook and stir until crisp-tender, about 4 minutes.

3. Add rice; cook and stir for 2 minutes. Add the broth mixture, a cup at a time, stirring until the liquid is absorbed, about 15 minutes. When there is 1 cup broth remaining, return the beef to the pot and add the steak sauce, pepper, and asparagus. Cook and stir until rice is tender, beef is cooked, and asparagus is tender, about 5 minutes. Stir in Parmesan and butter and serve immediately.

CALORIES: 365.04 | Fat: 11.67g | Saturated fat: 4.09g | Dietary fiber: 3.47g | Sodium: 138.81mg | Cholesterol: 36.20mg

Wasabi-Roasted Filet Mignon

Wasabi is like horseradish, but its flavor is much more intense.
It's served with sushi and other Japanese meals.

INGREDIENTS | SERVES 12

1 3-pound filet mignon roast

¼ teaspoon pepper

1 teaspoon powdered wasabi

2 tablespoons sesame oil

2 tablespoons soy sauce

Filet Mignon

Filet mignon is one of the most expensive cuts of steak, but it is almost 100 percent edible with no waste. The cut is very tender but not the most flavorful, so it is often cooked with very intense ingredients, like wasabi and jalapeño peppers. Slice it into very thin slices against the grain to serve.

1. Preheat oven to 400°F. If the roast has a thin end and a thick end, fold the thin end under so the roast is about the same thickness. Place on a roasting pan.

2. In a small bowl, combine pepper, wasabi, oil, and soy sauce, and mix well. Brush half over roast. Roast the beef for 30 minutes, then remove and brush with remaining wasabi mixture. Return to oven for 5–10 minutes longer or until meat thermometer registers at least 145°F for medium rare.

3. Remove from oven, cover, and let stand for 15 minutes before slicing to serve.

CALORIES: 298.15 | Fat: 24.00g | Saturated fat: 8.99g | Dietary fiber: 0.13g | Sodium: 143.07mg | Cholesterol: 68.57mg

Beef Rollups with Pesto

This recipe is perfect for entertaining. You can make the rollups ahead of time; don't dredge or brown them until about an hour before you'd like to eat.

INGREDIENTS | SERVES 6

½ cup packed basil leaves

½ cup packed baby spinach leaves

3 cloves garlic, minced

⅓ cup toasted chopped hazelnuts

⅛ teaspoon white pepper

2 tablespoons grated Parmesan cheese

2 tablespoons olive oil

2 tablespoons water

3 tablespoons flour

½ teaspoon paprika

6 4-ounce top round steaks, ¼" thick

2 oil-packed sun-dried tomatoes, minced

1 tablespoon canola oil

1 cup Low-Sodium Beef Broth (Chapter 16)

1. In a blender or food processor, combine basil, spinach, garlic, hazelnuts, and white pepper, and blend or process until finely chopped. Add Parmesan and blend again. Add olive oil and blend until a paste forms, then add water and blend.

2. On a shallow plate, combine flour and paprika and mix well. Place beef between sheets of waxed paper and pound until ⅛" thick. Spread pesto on one side of the pounded beef and sprinkle with tomatoes. Roll up, fastening closed with toothpicks.

3. Dredge rollups in flour mixture. Heat canola oil in large saucepan and brown rollups on all sides, about 5 minutes total. Pour beef broth into pan and bring to a simmer. Cover, reduce heat to low, and simmer for 40–50 minutes or until beef is tender.

CALORIES: 290.23 | Fat: 18.73g | Saturated fat: 3.90g | Dietary fiber: 1.03g | Sodium: 95.79mg | Cholesterol: 63.60mg

CHAPTER 18

Heart-Healthy Fish, Pasta, and Bean Main-Dish Recipes

Seafood Risotto

Risotto is an elegant dish, perfect for entertaining. Do all your prep work ahead of time and store ingredients in the fridge, and the dish will take only about 30 minutes of cooking time.

INGREDIENTS | SERVES 6

2 cups water

2½ cups Low-Sodium Chicken Broth (Chapter 16)

2 tablespoons olive oil

1 onion, minced

3 cloves garlic, minced

1½ cups Arborio rice

1 cup chopped celery

1 tablespoon fresh dill weed

¼ cup dry white wine

½ pound sole fillets

¼ pound small raw shrimp

½ pound bay scallops

¼ cup grated Parmesan cheese

1 tablespoon butter

1. In a medium saucepan, combine water and broth and heat over low heat. Keep mixture on heat.

2. In a large saucepan, heat olive oil over medium heat. Add onion and garlic; cook and stir until crisp-tender, about 3 minutes. Add rice; cook and stir for 3 minutes.

3. Start adding broth mixture, a cup at a time, stirring frequently, adding more liquid when the previous addition is absorbed. When only 1 cup of broth remains to be added, stir in celery, dill, wine, sole fillets, shrimp, and scallops to rice mixture. Add last cup of broth.

4. Cook, stirring constantly, for 5–7 minutes or until fish is cooked and rice is tender and creamy. Add Parmesan and butter, stir, and serve.

CALORIES: 397.22 | Fat: 11.11g | Saturated fat: 3.20g | Dietary fiber: 2.41g | Sodium: 354.58mg | Cholesterol: 94.39mg

Broiled Swordfish

This flavorful sauce and cooking method can be used with any fish.

INGREDIENTS | SERVES 4

1 tablespoon olive oil
2 tablespoons dry white wine
1 teaspoon lemon zest
¼ teaspoon salt
⅛ teaspoon white pepper
1 teaspoon dried dill weed
1¼ pounds swordfish steaks
4 ½"-thick tomato slices

1. Preheat broiler. In small bowl, combine oil, wine, zest, salt, pepper, and dill weed and whisk to blend.

2. Place steaks on a broiler pan. Brush steaks with oil mixture. Broil 6" from heat for 4 minutes. Turn fish over and brush with remaining oil mixture. Top with tomatoes. Return to broiler and broil for 4–6 minutes or until fish flakes when tested with a fork.

CALORIES: 210.97 | Fat: 9.10g | Saturated fat: 2.03g | Dietary fiber: 0.24g | Sodium: 273.91mg | Cholesterol: 55.25mg

Cajun-Rubbed Fish

Never marinate fish longer than 1 hour; otherwise, the flesh may become mushy.
This is a perfect last-minute dish for entertaining.

INGREDIENTS | SERVES 4

½ teaspoon black pepper
¼ teaspoon cayenne pepper
½ teaspoon lemon zest
½ teaspoon dried dill weed
⅛ teaspoon salt
1 tablespoon brown sugar
4 5-ounce swordfish steaks
Olive or vegetable oil, as needed

1. Prepare and preheat grill. In a small bowl, combine pepper, cayenne pepper, lemon zest, dill weed, salt, and brown sugar and mix well. Sprinkle onto both sides of the swordfish steaks and rub in. Set aside for 30 minutes.

2. Brush grill with oil. Add swordfish; cook without moving for 4 minutes. Carefully turn steaks and cook for 2–4 minutes on second side until fish just flakes when tested with fork. Serve immediately.

CALORIES: 233.57 | Fat: 7.31g | Saturated fat: 2.00g | Dietary fiber: 0.10g | Sodium: 237.08mg | Cholesterol: 70.83mg

Cod and Potatoes

*Thinly sliced potatoes are layered with olive oil and herbs and baked until crisp,
then topped with cod and lemon juice. Yum!*

INGREDIENTS | SERVES 4

3 Yukon Gold potatoes

¼ cup olive oil

⅛ teaspoon white pepper

1½ teaspoons dried herbes de Provence,
  divided

4 4-ounce cod steaks

1 tablespoon butter or margarine

2 tablespoons lemon juice

1. Preheat oven to 350°F. Spray a 9" glass baking dish with nonstick cooking spray. Thinly slice the potatoes. Layer in the baking dish, drizzling each layer with a tablespoon of olive oil, a sprinkle of pepper, and some of the herbes de Provence.

2. Bake for 30 minutes or until potatoes are browned on top and tender when pierced with a fork. Arrange cod steaks on top of potatoes. Dot with butter and sprinkle with lemon juice and remaining herbes de Provence.

3. Bake for 20 minutes longer or until fish flakes when tested with fork.

CALORIES: 362.62 | Fat: 17.28g | Saturated fat: 3.88g | Dietary fiber: 3.55g | Sodium: 91.56mg | Cholesterol: 56.36mg

Baked Lemon Sole with Herbed Crumbs

*Adding herbs to bread crumbs is a wonderful way to make a
flavorful crust on fish without adding calories, fat, or sodium.*

INGREDIENTS | SERVES 4

2 slices Light Whole-Grain Bread
  (Chapter 19), crumbled

2 tablespoons minced parsley

2 cloves garlic, minced

1 teaspoon dried dill weed

2 tablespoons olive oil

4 6-ounce sole fillets

2 tablespoons lemon juice

Pinch salt

⅛ teaspoon white pepper

1. Preheat oven to 350°F. In a small bowl, combine bread crumbs, parsley, garlic, and dill weed, and mix well. Drizzle with olive oil and toss to coat.

2. Spray a 9" baking dish with nonstick cooking spray and arrange fillets in dish. Sprinkle with lemon juice, salt, and pepper. Divide crumb mixture on top of fillets.

3. Bake for 15 minutes or until fish flakes when tested with a fork and crumb topping is browned. Serve immediately.

CALORIES: 294.58 | Fat: 9.86g | Saturated fat: 1.65g | Dietary fiber: 1.09g | Sodium: 288.21mg | Cholesterol: 110.78mg

Salmon Vegetable Stir-Fry

Sturdy vegetables are used in this stir-fry because they can continue cooking while the salmon steams.

INGREDIENTS | SERVES 4

2 tablespoons rice vinegar

1 tablespoon sugar

1 tablespoon grated gingerroot

1 tablespoon cornstarch

2 tablespoons hoisin sauce

⅛ teaspoon white pepper

2 tablespoons peanut oil

1 onion, sliced

½ pound sugar-snap peas

3 carrots, sliced

1 red bell pepper, sliced

¾ pound salmon fillet

Hoisin Sauce

Hoisin sauce is used in Asian cooking. It's a rich, thick, dark, and sweet sauce that stands up to the rich flavors of salmon. It is used sparingly, usually mixed into a stir-fry sauce or marinade. Hoisin sauce is made from fermented soybeans, vinegar, sugar, garlic, and chili peppers.

1. In small bowl, combine rice vinegar, sugar, gingerroot, cornstarch, hoisin sauce, and pepper. Mix well and set aside.

2. In large skillet or wok, heat peanut oil over high heat. Add onion, peas, and carrots. Stir-fry for 3–4 minutes or until vegetables begin to soften. Add red bell pepper.

3. Immediately place salmon fillet on top of vegetables. Reduce heat to medium, cover skillet or wok and cook for 4–5 minutes or until salmon flakes when tested with fork.

4. Stir the vinegar mixture and add to skillet or wok. Turn heat to medium-high and stir-fry to break up the salmon for 2–3 minutes until the sauce bubbles and thickens. Serve immediately over hot cooked rice.

CALORIES: 371.71 | Fat: 11.73g | Saturated fat: 3.24g | Dietary fiber: 4.51g | Sodium: 237.60mg | Cholesterol: 67.11mg

Seared Scallops with Fruit

Serve this super-quick and colorful dish with brown-rice pilaf and a green salad.

INGREDIENTS | SERVES 3–4

1 pound sea scallops

Pinch salt

⅛ teaspoon white pepper

1 tablespoon olive oil

1 tablespoon butter or margarine

2 peaches, sliced

¼ cup dry white wine

1 cup blueberries

1 tablespoon lime juice

1. Rinse scallops and pat dry. Sprinkle with salt and pepper and set aside.

2. In large skillet, heat olive oil and butter over medium-high heat. Add the scallops and don't move them for 3 minutes. When the scallops turn deep golden-brown, turn and cook for 1–2 minutes on the second side.

3. Remove scallops to serving plate. Add peaches to skillet and brown quickly on one side. Turn peaches and add wine to skillet; bring to a boil. Remove from heat and add blueberries. Pour over scallops, sprinkle with lime juice, and serve immediately.

CALORIES: 207.89 | Fat: 7.36g | Saturated fat: 2.40g | Dietary fiber: 1.62g | Sodium: 242.16mg | Cholesterol: 45.03mg

Pistachio-Crusted Red Snapper

This could also be made with other heart-healthy nuts, including hazelnuts, walnuts, or pecans.

INGREDIENTS | SERVES 4

1 tablespoon lemon juice

1 teaspoon grated orange zest

1 teaspoon grated lemon zest

2 tablespoons olive oil

⅓ cup chopped pistachios

1 slice Light Whole-Grain Bread (Chapter 19), crumbled

1 pound red snapper fillets

Pinch salt

⅛ teaspoon pepper

1. Preheat oven to 375°F. In a bowl, combine lemon juice, orange zest, lemon zest, and olive oil. In another bowl, combine chopped pistachios and crumbled bread. Drizzle lemon mixture over bread mixture and toss to coat.

2. Spray a 9"-square glass baking dish with nonstick cooking spray. Arrange fish in dish and sprinkle with salt and pepper. Top evenly with the crumb mixture.

3. Bake for 20 minutes, or until fish is opaque and flakes when tested with fork and crumb mixture is browned. Serve immediately.

CALORIES: 283.52 | Fat: 15.79g | Saturated fat: 2.20g | Dietary fiber: 2.29g | Sodium: 172.06mg | Cholesterol: 54.40mg

Sesame-Crusted Mahi Mahi

The sesame seeds toast while the fish cooks, and the mustard mixture seals in the moisture in this fabulously easy recipe.

INGREDIENTS | SERVES 4

4 4-ounce mahi mahi or sole fillets
2 tablespoons Dijon mustard
1 tablespoon low-fat sour cream
½ cup sesame seeds
2 tablespoons olive oil
1 lemon, cut into wedges

1. Rinse fillets and pat dry. In a small bowl, combine mustard and sour cream and mix well. Spread this mixture on all sides of fish. Roll in sesame seeds to coat.

2. Heat olive oil in large skillet over medium heat. Pan-fry fish, turning once, for 5–8 minutes or until fish flakes when tested with fork and sesame seeds are toasted. Serve immediately with lemon wedges.

CALORIES: 282.75 | Fat: 17.17g | Saturated fat: 2.84g | Dietary fiber: 2.42g | Sodium: 209.54mg | Cholesterol: 73.75mg

Scallops on Skewers with Tomatoes

This sauce is a variation on chimichurri sauce, originally from Argentina. It's fragrant and delicious.

INGREDIENTS | SERVES 4

1 pound sea scallops
12 cherry tomatoes
4 green onions, cut in half crosswise
½ cup chopped parsley
1 tablespoon fresh oregano leaves
3 tablespoons olive oil
2 tablespoons lemon juice
2 cloves garlic
⅛ teaspoon salt
⅛ teaspoon pepper

1. Prepare and preheat broiler. Rinse scallops and pat dry. Thread on skewers along with cherry tomatoes and green onions.

2. In a blender or food processor, combine remaining ingredients. Blend or process until smooth. Reserve ¼ cup of this sauce.

3. Brush remaining sauce onto the food on the skewers. Place on broiler pan. Broil 6" from heat for 3–4 minutes per side, turning once during cooking time. Serve with remaining sauce.

CALORIES: 202.03 | Fat: 11.11g | Saturated fat: 1.52g | Dietary fiber: 1.34g | Sodium: 251.50mg | Cholesterol: 35.06mg

Sesame-Pepper Salmon Kabobs

Serve these skewers on brown-rice pilaf with a wedge of lemon on the side.
A fruit salad will round out the meal.

INGREDIENTS | SERVES 4

1 pound salmon steak
2 tablespoons olive oil, divided
¼ cup sesame seeds
1 teaspoon pepper
1 red bell pepper
1 yellow bell pepper
1 red onion
8 cremini mushrooms
⅛ teaspoon salt

1. Prepare and preheat grill. Cut salmon steak into 1" pieces, discarding skin and bones. Brush salmon with half of the olive oil.

2. In a small bowl, combine sesame seeds and pepper and mix. Press all sides of salmon cubes into the sesame seed mixture.

3. Slice bell peppers into 1" slices and cut red onion into 8 wedges; trim mushroom stems and leave caps whole. Skewer coated salmon pieces, peppers, onion, and mushrooms on metal skewers. Brush vegetables with remaining olive oil and sprinkle with salt.

4. Grill 6" from medium coals, turning once during cooking time, until the sesame seeds are very brown and toasted and fish is just done, about 6–8 minutes. Serve immediately.

CALORIES: 319.33 | Fat: 20.26g | Saturated fat: 3.67g | Dietary fiber: 2.39g | Sodium: 141.88mg | Cholesterol: 66.94mg

Almond Snapper with Shrimp Sauce

You could use any mild white fish in this delicious recipe.

INGREDIENTS | SERVES 6

1 egg white

¼ cup dry bread crumbs

⅓ cup ground almonds

⅛ teaspoon salt

⅛ teaspoon white pepper

6 4-ounce red snapper fillets

3 tablespoons olive oil

1 onion, chopped

4 cloves garlic, minced

1 red bell pepper, chopped

¼ pound small raw shrimp, deshelled and deveined

1 tablespoon lemon juice

½ cup low-fat sour cream

½ teaspoon dried dill weed

1. Place egg white in a shallow bowl; beat until foamy. On a shallow plate, combine bread crumbs, almonds, salt, and pepper and mix well. Dip fish into egg white, then into crumb mixture, pressing to coat. Let stand on a wire rack for 10 minutes.

2. In a small saucepan, heat 1 tablespoon olive oil over medium heat. Add onion, garlic, and bell pepper; cook and stir until tender, about 5 minutes. Add shrimp; cook and stir just until shrimp curl and turn pink, about 1–2 minutes. Remove from heat and add lemon juice; set aside.

3. In a large saucepan, heat remaining 2 tablespoons olive oil over medium heat. Add coated fish fillets. Cook for 4 minutes on one side, then carefully turn and cook for 2–5 minutes on second side until coating is browned and fish flakes when tested with a fork.

4. While fish is cooking, return saucepan with shrimp to medium heat. Add sour cream and dill weed. Heat, stirring, until mixture is hot.

5. Remove fish from skillet and place on serving plate. Top each with a spoonful of shrimp sauce and serve immediately.

CALORIES: 272.57 | Fat: 13.80g | Saturated fat: 3.09g | Dietary fiber: 1.56g | Sodium: 216.17mg | Cholesterol: 88.71mg

Scallops on Skewers with Lemon

*Because scallops are so low in fat, sodium, and cholesterol,
you can add a bit of low-sodium bacon to this dish for a flavor treat.*

INGREDIENTS | SERVES 4

2 tablespoons lemon juice

1 teaspoon grated lemon zest

2 teaspoons sesame oil

2 tablespoons chili sauce

⅛ teaspoon cayenne pepper

1 pound sea scallops

4 strips low-sodium bacon

Bacon

If you read labels and choose carefully, you can have bacon as an occasional treat. Many companies now make low-sodium bacon. In health-food stores you can often find organic bacon that has better nutrition. Also consider Canadian bacon. More like ham, this meat has less sodium, fat, and chemicals like nitrates than regular bacon.

1. Prepare and preheat grill or broiler. In a medium bowl, combine lemon juice, zest, sesame oil, chili sauce, and cayenne pepper and mix well. Add scallops and toss to coat. Let stand for 15 minutes.

2. Make skewers with the scallops and bacon. Thread a skewer through one end of the bacon, then add a scallop. Curve the bacon around the scallop and thread onto the skewer so it surrounds the scallop halfway. Repeat with 3 to 4 more scallops and the bacon slice.

3. Repeat with remaining scallops and bacon. Grill or broil 6" from heat source for 3–5 minutes per side, until bacon is crisp and scallops are cooked and opaque. Serve immediately.

CALORIES: 173.65 | Fat: 6.48g | Saturated fat: 1.51g | Dietary fiber: 0.07g | Sodium: 266.64mg | Cholesterol: 46.20mg

Spaghetti Sauce

Grated carrots add nutrition and fiber to this rich sauce and help reduce the problem of sauce separation.

INGREDIENTS | YIELDS 6 CUPS; SERVING SIZE 1 CUP

2 tablespoons olive oil

1 onion, chopped

4 cloves garlic, minced

1 cup chopped celery

1 8-ounce package sliced mushrooms

1 6-ounce can no-salt tomato paste

2 14-ounce cans no-salt diced tomatoes, undrained

1 tablespoon dried Italian seasoning

½ cup grated carrots

⅛ teaspoon white pepper

½ cup dry red wine

½ cup water

1. In a large saucepan, heat olive oil over medium heat. Add onion and garlic; cook and stir until crisp-tender, about 4 minutes. Add celery and mushrooms; cook and stir for 2–3 minutes longer.

2. Add tomato paste; let paste brown a bit without stirring (this adds flavor to the sauce). Then add remaining ingredients and stir gently but thoroughly.

3. Bring sauce to a simmer, then reduce heat to low and partially cover. Simmer for 60–70 minutes, stirring occasionally, until sauce is blended and thickened. Serve over hot cooked pasta, couscous, or rice.

CALORIES: 155.73 | Fat: 5.11g | Saturated fat: 0.72g | Dietary fiber: 4.96g | Sodium: 84.74mg | Cholesterol: 0.0g

Freezing Spaghetti Sauce

Spaghetti sauce freezes beautifully, and it is suitable for all sorts of casseroles and soups in addition to just serving it over spaghetti. To freeze, portion 4 cups into a hard-sided freezer container, leaving about 1" of head space for expansion. Seal, label, and freeze for up to 3 months. To thaw, let stand in fridge overnight, then heat in saucepan.

Spaghetti with Creamy Tomato Sauce

You can serve this simple and flavorful recipe to just about anybody!

INGREDIENTS | SERVES 6–8

1 recipe Spaghetti Sauce (see previous recipe)

½ cup fat-free half-and-half

1 16-ounce package whole-grain pasta

½ cup grated Parmesan cheese

Tomatoes

Tomatoes are an excellent heart-healthy food, high in vitamins C and A and with no fat or cholesterol. They are usually sold unripe in the supermarket. Let them stand at room temperature for 1–2 days until they give to slight pressure. Don't store tomatoes in the refrigerator; their texture will become mealy.

1. Bring large pot of water to a boil. Prepare Spaghetti Sauce as directed. During last 5 minutes of cooking time, add half-and-half and stir to blend.

2. Cook pasta in boiling water according to package directions until al dente. Drain and add to Spaghetti Sauce; cook and stir for 1 minute to let the pasta absorb some of the sauce. Sprinkle with Parmesan and serve immediately.

CALORIES: 354.63 | Fat: 6.65g | Saturated fat: 1.90g | Dietary fiber: 3.90g | Sodium: 188.68mg | Cholesterol: 6.26mg

Chickpeas in Lettuce Wraps

This delicious creamy and flavorful spread is also great spread on toasted bread or used as an appetizer dip.

INGREDIENTS | SERVES 6–8

1 15-ounce can no-salt chickpeas

3 tablespoons olive oil

3 tablespoons lemon juice

3 cloves garlic, minced

1 tablespoon chopped fresh mint

½ cup diced red onion

8 lettuce leaves

1 cup chopped tomatoes

1 cup chopped yellow bell pepper

1. Drain the chickpeas; rinse, and drain again. Place half in a blender or food processor. Add olive oil, lemon juice, garlic, and mint. Blend or process until smooth.

2. Place in a medium bowl and stir in remaining chickpeas and red onion; stir until combined.

3. To make the wraps, place lettuce leaves on work surface. Divide chickpea mixture among leaves and top with tomatoes and bell pepper. Roll up, folding in sides, to enclose filling. Serve immediately.

CALORIES: 148.96 | Fat: 6.56g | Saturated fat: 0.87g | Dietary fiber: 4.98g | Sodium: 6.80g | Cholesterol: 0.0g

Pasta Salad with Crunchy Vegetables

Any fresh vegetables that are typically eaten raw would be delicious in this flavorful salad; you could add mushrooms, other bell peppers, or zucchini.

INGREDIENTS | SERVES 8

½ cup low-fat mayonnaise

⅓ cup olive oil

¼ cup white wine vinegar

2 cloves garlic, minced

1 teaspoon chopped fresh oregano

¼ cup chopped flat-leaf parsley

⅛ teaspoon pepper

2 red bell peppers, chopped

4 stalks celery, chopped

1 yellow summer squash, chopped

1 pint grape tomatoes

1 16-ounce package whole-grain rotini pasta

1. Bring a large pot of water to a boil. In a large bowl, combine mayonnaise, olive oil, vinegar, garlic, oregano, parsley, and pepper and mix well with wire whisk to blend.

2. Stir in bell peppers, celery, squash, and tomatoes, and mix well. Cook pasta according to package directions until al dente. Drain and immediately add to salad in bowl. Stir gently to coat pasta with dressing. Cover and refrigerate for 4 hours before serving.

CALORIES: 362.47 | Fat: 15.12g | Saturated fat: 2.21g | Dietary fiber: 1.80g | Sodium: 131.65mg | Cholesterol: 0.0mg

Whole-Grain Pasta

If you're avoiding simple carbohydrates, whole-grain pastas are a wonderful way to start eating pasta again. These pastas are readily available in the local grocery store. They have a stronger flavor than plain pastas, so you may want to mix the two kinds half-and-half at first to introduce whole-grain pasta to your family.

CHAPTER 19

Heart-Healthy Bread, Dessert, and Dressing Recipes

Chocolate Pancakes

Chocolate pancakes are a nice treat for breakfast or brunch.
Serve them with warmed maple syrup or whipped honey.

INGREDIENTS | SERVES 6–8

1½ cups flour

⅓ cup sugar

1 teaspoon baking powder

½ teaspoon baking soda

¼ cup cocoa powder

½ teaspoon salt

¼ cup vegetable oil

1 egg

1 egg white

½ cup buttermilk

1 teaspoon vanilla

2 tablespoons butter or margarine

Baking Powder

Look for baking powder that uses phosphates, not aluminum, for your baking and cooking needs. This type has no harsh aftertaste. It's sold in large grocery and health-food stores. But make sure that the baking powder you buy is double-acting. This means that it reacts with liquid when first mixed with the batter to form CO_2 and forms more CO_2 when heated.

1. In a medium bowl, combine flour, sugar, baking powder, baking soda, cocoa, and salt. In small bowl, combine oil, egg, egg white, buttermilk, and vanilla and beat until blended.

2. Add wet ingredients to dry ingredients and mix just until smooth, using an eggbeater or wire whisk. Let stand for 10 minutes.

3. Heat a large griddle or frying pan over medium heat. Grease the griddle with some of the butter. Pour batter in ¼-cup portions onto griddle. Cook until the sides look dry and bubbles begin to form and break on the surface, about 3–5 minutes. Turn and cook for 1–2 minutes on second side; serve immediately.

CALORIES: 227.12 | Fat: 11.05g | Saturated fat: 3.23g | Dietary fiber: 1.53g | Sodium: 177.18mg | Cholesterol: 34.68mg

Vegetable Omelet

You could use other vegetables in this colorful omelet. Chopped mushrooms, summer squash, or bell pepper are delicious possibilities.

INGREDIENTS | SERVES 4

1 tablespoon olive oil

½ cup grated carrot

½ cup chopped broccoli

¼ cup finely chopped red onion

8 egg whites

1 egg yolk

¼ cup 1% milk

⅛ teaspoon white pepper

½ cup grated extra-sharp Cheddar cheese

1. In large nonstick skillet, heat olive oil over medium heat. Add carrot, broccoli, and onion; cook, stirring occasionally, until crisp-tender, about 4–5 minutes.

2. Meanwhile, in medium bowl, beat egg whites until a soft foam forms. In small bowl, combine egg yolk with milk and pepper and beat well. Fold egg-yolk mixture into egg whites.

3. Pour the egg mixture into the pan. Cook, lifting the edges of the eggs so the uncooked mixture can flow underneath, until eggs are set but still moist. Sprinkle with cheese and cover pan; cook for 1 minute. Uncover, fold omelet, and serve immediately.

CALORIES: 156.08 | Fat: 9.54g | Saturated fat: 3.96g | Dietary fiber: 1.11g | Sodium: 220.56mg | Cholesterol: 68.04mg

Cinnamon Granola

Homemade granola makes not only a great breakfast but a fabulous snack, too. And you can sprinkle it on frozen yogurt or sherbet for a super-quick dessert.

INGREDIENTS | SERVES 16; SERVING SIZE ½ CUP

4 cups regular oats

¼ cup oat bran

¼ cup flaxseed

1 cup chopped walnuts

½ cup honey

¼ cup brown sugar

3 tablespoons orange juice

¼ cup canola oil

¼ teaspoon salt

1 tablespoon vanilla

1 tablespoon cinnamon

1 cup dried sweetened cranberries

1 cup raisins

Flaxseed

You can find flaxseed in health-food stores and co-ops, as well as online. Also at these locations you can find flaxseed oil for use in baking and cooking. Flaxseed contains lignans, a type of soluble fiber, and alpha linolenic acids, similar to omega-3 fatty acids, which can lower total LDL cholesterol and help prevent blood platelets from sticking together.

1. Preheat oven to 300°F. Spray a cookie sheet with sides with nonstick cooking spray and set aside.

2. In large bowl, combine oats, oat bran, flaxseed, and walnuts and mix well. In small saucepan, combine honey, sugar, orange juice, canola oil, and salt and heat over low heat until warm. Remove from heat and add vanilla.

3. Pour honey mixture over oat mixture and mix well until oat mixture is coated. Spoon onto prepared cookie sheet and spread into an even layer.

4. Bake granola for 45 minutes, stirring every 10 minutes. Remove from oven, sprinkle with cinnamon, and stir in cranberries and raisins. Cool completely, then store in airtight container at room temperature.

CALORIES: 357.05 | Fat: 11.14g | Saturated fat: 1.03g | Dietary fiber: 7.01g | Sodium: 78.62mg | Cholesterol: 0.0mg

Whole-Grain Waffles

Homemade waffles taste so much better than frozen.
You can use them for breakfast with fresh fruit, or serve them for dinner with some chili.

INGREDIENTS | SERVES 8

1 cup all-purpose flour

¾ cup whole-wheat flour

1 cup cornmeal

2 teaspoons baking powder

½ teaspoon baking soda

⅛ teaspoon salt

1 egg

2 tablespoons butter or margarine, melted

2 cups buttermilk

4 egg whites

¼ cup sugar

Waffles

The first waffle you cook almost always sticks; you can consider it a test waffle. Lightly spray the waffle iron with nonstick cooking spray before you add the batter each time, and remove any bits of the previous waffle before adding batter. You might need nonstick cooking spray with flour as extra protection against sticking.

1. In a medium bowl, combine all-purpose flour, whole-wheat flour, cornmeal, baking powder, baking soda, and salt, and mix well.

2. In a small bowl, combine egg, melted butter, and buttermilk and mix well. Add to flour mixture and stir just until combined.

3. In a large bowl, beat egg whites until foamy. Gradually add sugar, beating until stiff peaks form. Fold into flour mixture.

4. Spray a waffle iron with nonstick cooking spray and heat according to directions. Pour about ¼ cup batter into the waffle iron, close, and cook until the steaming stops, or according to the appliance directions. Serve immediately.

CALORIES: 250.62 | Fat: 4.71g | Saturated fat: 2.45g | Dietary fiber: 3.07g | Sodium: 291.70mg | Cholesterol: 36.51mg

Buckwheat Pancakes

Because buckwheat is a fruit, not a grain, buckwheat flour is gluten-free. It is high in protein and fiber, making it a good choice for people watching their cholesterol.

INGREDIENTS | SERVES 4

½ cup buttermilk

2 tablespoons butter or margarine, melted

2 egg whites

½ cup buckwheat flour

½ cup all-purpose flour

1½ teaspoons baking powder

½ teaspoon baking soda

3 tablespoons sugar

Nonstick cooking spray

1. In bowl, combine buttermilk, butter, and egg whites, and beat well. Set aside.

2. In large bowl, combine buckwheat flour, all-purpose flour, baking powder, baking soda, and sugar and mix well. Form a well in the center of the dry ingredients and add the wet ingredients. Stir just until batter is mixed; do not overmix.

3. Spray a skillet with nonstick cooking spray and heat over medium heat. Using a ¼-cup measure, pour four pancakes at once onto the griddle. Cook until bubbles form on the surface and begin to break. Flip pancakes and cook for 1–2 minutes on second side. Serve immediately.

CALORIES: 215.98 | Fat: 6.67g | Saturated fat: 3.94g | Dietary fiber: 1.93g | Sodium: 350.46mg | Cholesterol: 16.48mg

Blueberry Corn Pancakes

The combination of sweet roasted corn with tart blueberries is really wonderful.
Serve with warmed blueberry or maple syrup.

INGREDIENTS | SERVES 6

1 cup frozen corn

1 tablespoon olive oil

1¼ cups all-purpose flour

¼ cup cornmeal

2 teaspoons baking powder

3 tablespoons sugar

1 egg

2 egg whites

¼ cup buttermilk

¼ cup orange juice

2 tablespoons butter or margarine, melted

1 teaspoon grated orange zest

½ cup fresh or frozen blueberries

About Pancakes

Pancakes are easy, if you follow a few rules. First of all, don't overmix the batter; there should be a few lumps. When you cook the pancakes, pour the batter onto the hot griddle, then don't touch it until the sides start to look dry and bubbles form on the surface of the pancake. Carefully flip the pancakes and cook for another couple of minutes.

1. Preheat oven to 400°F. Place corn on a small cookie sheet and drizzle with olive oil. Roast for 15–25 minutes or until corn begins to turn golden-brown on the edges. Remove from oven and cool completely.

2. In a large bowl, combine flour, cornmeal, baking powder, and sugar and mix well. In small bowl, combine egg, egg whites, buttermilk, orange juice, melted butter, and orange zest and beat until combined.

3. Stir egg mixture into flour mixture just until combined, then fold in cooled corn and blueberries.

4. Heat a large skillet or griddle. Spray with nonstick cooking spray. Pour batter by ¼-cup portions onto skillet, making four pancakes at a time. Cook until bubbles form on the surface and begin to break, about 2–4 minutes. Carefully turn pancakes and cook for 1–2 minutes on the second side. Serve immediately.

CALORIES: 225.39 | Fat: 5.36g | Saturated fat: 2.83g | Dietary fiber: 1.81g | Sodium: 190.53mg | Cholesterol: 45.83mg

Blueberry-Banana Smoothie

Smoothies are a great way to eat breakfast on the run, but they can have lots of calories.
Use nonfat ingredients, and pile on the fruit!

INGREDIENTS | SERVES 2

1½ cups skim milk

1 banana

1 cup blueberries

1 cup nonfat vanilla yogurt

4 ice cubes

Place milk, banana, blueberries, and yogurt in blender or food processor; blend or process until smooth. Add ice cubes; blend or process until thick. Pour into glasses and serve immediately.

CALORIES: 283.52 | Fat: 4.83g | Saturated fat: 2.77g | Dietary fiber: 3.51g | Sodium: 159.60mg | Cholesterol: 5.12mg

Blueberries

Blueberries are one of the healthiest foods on the planet. Their antioxidant count is through the roof. In fact, blueberries lower cholesterol better than statin drugs! Add a cup of blueberries a day to your diet to really improve your health.

PB&J Smoothies

Remember, peanut butter is cholesterol-free because it is made from plant materials.
You can find low-fat versions of peanut butter on the market.

INGREDIENTS | SERVES 3

1 cup raspberry yogurt

1 cup skim milk

3 tablespoons peanut butter

½ cup frozen vanilla yogurt

2 tablespoons raspberry jelly

In blender or food processor, combine yogurt, milk, peanut butter, and frozen yogurt. Blend or process until smooth. By hand, stir in the jelly just until marbled. Pour into glasses and serve immediately.

CALORIES: 238.61 | Fat: 9.89g | Saturated fat: 2.47g | Dietary fiber: 1.42g | Sodium: 92.47mg | Cholesterol: 3.62mg

Orange-Vanilla Smoothie

You can vary this smoothie in so many ways. Use pineapple yogurt, pineapple nectar, and crushed pineapple instead of the orange. Use your imagination!

INGREDIENTS | SERVES 2

1½ cups orange yogurt

½ cup orange juice

1 orange, peeled and sliced

¼ cup vanilla-flavored whey protein

1 teaspoon vanilla

4 ice cubes

Place yogurt, orange juice, orange, whey protein, and vanilla in blender or food processor; blend or process until smooth. Add ice cubes; blend or process until thick. Pour into glasses and serve immediately.

CALORIES: 346.91 | Fat: 2.34g | Saturated fat: 1.22g | Dietary fiber: 2.33g | Sodium: 241.12mg | Cholesterol: 6.81mg

Apple-Cinnamon Smoothie

Applesauce is available in several versions; you can find chunky applesauce, smooth applesauce, and organic applesauce.

INGREDIENTS | SERVES 2

1 cup applesauce

½ cup vanilla yogurt

½ teaspoon cinnamon

1 apple, peeled and chopped

4 ice cubes

Place applesauce, yogurt, cinnamon, and apple in blender or food processor; blend or process until smooth. Add ice cubes; blend or process until thick. Pour into glasses and serve immediately.

CALORIES: 179.68 | Fat: 1.08g | Saturated fat: 0.55g | Dietary fiber: 2.36g | Sodium: 44.25mg | Cholesterol: 3.06mg

Banana-Blueberry Oatmeal Bread

Quick breads are easy to make. Their flavor and texture usually gets better if allowed to stand, covered, overnight at room temperature.

INGREDIENTS | YIELDS 1 LOAF; 12 SERVINGS

1 3-ounce package light cream cheese, softened

¼ cup brown sugar

¼ cup sugar

2 bananas, mashed

1 egg

2 egg whites

¼ cup orange juice

1 cup all-purpose flour

½ cup whole-wheat flour

1 teaspoon baking powder

1 teaspoon baking soda

1 cup blueberries

½ cup regular oatmeal

1. Preheat oven to 350°F. Spray a 9" × 5" loaf pan with nonstick cooking spray containing flour, and set aside.

2. In a large bowl, combine cream cheese with brown sugar and sugar and beat until fluffy. Beat in mashed bananas, then add egg, egg whites, and orange juice and beat until smooth.

3. Stir together all-purpose flour, whole-wheat flour, baking powder, and baking soda. Add to batter and stir just until combined. Fold in blueberries and oatmeal. Pour into prepared loaf pan.

4. Bake for 50–60 minutes or until bread is deep golden-brown and a toothpick inserted in the center comes out clean. Remove from pan and cool on a wire rack.

CALORIES: 165.78 | Fat: 2.43g | Saturated fat: 1.05g | Dietary fiber: 2.39g | Sodium: 173.82mg | Cholesterol: 21.59mg

Fresh or Frozen Fruit?

When baking, you can usually use either fresh or frozen fruit. If using frozen fruit, do not thaw before adding it to the batter, or it will add too much liquid and color or stain the bread. Use frozen fruits that are dry-packed, with no added sugar or other ingredients.

Zucchini-Walnut Bread

When your garden is overflowing with zucchini in late summer, make several batches of this bread and freeze for the long winter months.

INGREDIENTS | YIELDS 1 LOAF; 12 SERVINGS

¼ cup canola oil

¼ cup sugar

½ cup brown sugar

1 egg

2 egg whites

½ cup orange juice

2 teaspoons vanilla

1 cup grated zucchini

1 teaspoon grated lemon zest

2 tablespoons wheat germ

1 cup all-purpose flour

1 cup whole-wheat flour

1 teaspoon baking powder

½ teaspoon baking soda

⅛ teaspoon salt

1 teaspoon cinnamon

¼ teaspoon cloves

½ cup chopped walnuts

1. Preheat oven to 350°F. Spray a 9" × 5" loaf pan with nonstick cooking spray containing flour, and set aside.

2. In large bowl, combine oil, sugar, brown sugar, egg, egg whites, orange juice, and vanilla and beat until smooth. Stir in zucchini, lemon zest, and wheat germ.

3. Sift together all-purpose flour, whole-wheat flour, baking powder, baking soda, salt, cinnamon, and cloves, and add to oil mixture. Stir just until combined, then fold in walnuts. Pour into prepared pan.

4. Bake for 55–65 minutes or until bread is golden-brown and a toothpick inserted in center comes out clean. Remove from pan and let cool on a wire rack.

CALORIES: 217.46 | Fat: 8.48g | Saturated fat: 0.70g | Dietary fiber: 2.13g | Sodium: 127.63mg | Cholesterol: 17.63mg

Fruity Oatmeal Coffee Cake

This coffee cake is full of fruit, oatmeal, and nuts. It's delicious served still warm from the oven.

INGREDIENTS | SERVES 16

½ cup brown sugar

1½ teaspoons cinnamon

1 cup oatmeal

½ cup chopped walnuts

6 tablespoons canola oil

2 tablespoons butter or plant sterol margarine

1 cup blueberries

½ cup dried cranberries

1 egg

2 egg whites

¾ cup buttermilk

¼ cup orange juice

⅔ cup sugar

1 cup all-purpose flour

1 cup whole-wheat flour

2 teaspoons baking powder

1 teaspoon baking soda

1. Preheat oven to 350°F. Spray a 13" × 9" baking pan with nonstick cooking spray containing flour, and set aside.

2. In a medium bowl, combine brown sugar, cinnamon, oatmeal, and walnuts and mix well. In a small saucepan, melt together 2 tablespoons canola oil and the butter. Pour into oatmeal mixture and stir until crumbs form. Add blueberries and cranberries; set aside.

3. In a large bowl, combine remaining 4 tablespoons oil, egg, egg whites, buttermilk, orange juice, and sugar and beat until combined. Add all-purpose flour, whole-wheat flour, baking powder, and baking soda and stir just until dry ingredients are moistened.

4. Spoon and spread batter into the prepared pan. Evenly sprinkle oatmeal mixture over the batter. Bake for 30–40 minutes or until coffee cake is golden-brown and a toothpick inserted in center comes out clean. Serve warm.

CALORIES: 261.93 | Fat: 10.24g | Saturated fat: 1.72g | Dietary fiber: 2.96g | Sodium: 161.27mg | Cholesterol: 17.49mg

Applesauce Cinnamon Bread

If you don't want to use liquid egg substitute, use 1 egg and 2 egg whites.

INGREDIENTS | YIELDS 1 LOAF; 12 SERVINGS

1¼ cups applesauce

1 cup brown sugar, divided

⅓ cup canola oil

¼ cup skim milk

½ cup liquid egg substitute

1 cup all-purpose flour

¾ cup whole-wheat flour

2 tablespoons wheat germ

1½ teaspoons cinnamon, divided

½ teaspoon nutmeg

1 teaspoon baking powder

½ teaspoon baking soda

½ cup golden raisins

½ cup chopped walnuts

Wheat Germ

Wheat germ is very high in fiber and anti-oxidants. It's made from the kernel of the grain. Its vitamin-E content can help reduce oxidation of cholesterol in your blood, thus reducing the risk of plaque formation. Wheat germ is also high in oil and can go rancid quite quickly. For the longest life, store it in the refrigerator.

1. Preheat oven to 350°F. Spray a 9" × 5" loaf pan with nonstick cooking spray containing flour, and set aside.

2. In a large bowl, combine applesauce, ¾ cup plus 2 tablespoons brown sugar, canola oil, milk, and egg substitute and beat well.

3. In a medium bowl, combine all-purpose flour, whole-wheat flour, wheat germ, 1 teaspoon cinnamon, nutmeg, baking powder, baking soda, raisins, and walnuts, and mix well. Add to applesauce mixture and stir until combined.

4. Pour batter into the prepared pan. In small bowl, combine remaining 2 tablespoons brown sugar with remaining ½ teaspoon cinnamon and mix well. Sprinkle evenly over batter in pan. Bake for 55–65 minutes or until bread is golden-brown and a toothpick inserted in center comes out clean. Remove from pan and let cool on a wire rack.

CALORIES: 263.33 | Fat: 9.88g | Saturated fat: 0.75g | Dietary fiber: 2.24g | Sodium: 113.09mg | Cholesterol: 0.21mg

Mixed-Nut Spice Muffins

Nuts are an important part of a cholesterol-reducing diet.
These spicy muffins are easy, perfect for breakfast on the run.

INGREDIENTS | YIELDS 12 MUFFINS

¼ cup canola oil

½ cup apricot jam

1 egg

2 egg whites

3 tablespoons lemon juice

½ cup orange juice

2 cups all-purpose flour

1½ teaspoons baking powder

⅛ teaspoon salt

1 teaspoon cinnamon

¼ teaspoon nutmeg

¼ teaspoon allspice

½ cup chopped hazelnuts, toasted

¼ cup chopped macadamia nuts,
  toasted

¼ cup chopped walnuts, toasted

1. Preheat oven to 400°F. Line 12 muffin cups with paper liners and set aside.

2. In a large bowl, combine oil, jam, egg, egg whites, lemon juice, and orange juice and whisk to blend. Add remaining ingredients and stir until just combined.

3. Fill each prepared muffin cup three-quarters full. Bake for 18–24 minutes or until muffins are set and golden-brown. Remove from muffin cups immediately and cool on a wire rack.

CALORIES: 229.28 | Fat: 11.80g | Saturated fat: 1.12g | Dietary fiber: 1.50g | Sodium: 90.32mg | Cholesterol: 17.62mg

Toasting Nuts

Toasting nuts brings out their flavor so you use less of them. To toast nuts, spread in a single layer on a baking or cookie sheet. Bake in a preheated 350°F oven for 8–12 minutes, stirring twice during cooking time, until the nuts turn a darker color and are fragrant. You can also toast them in a dry skillet for 4–6 minutes. Let cool completely before chopping.

Good-Morning Muffins

These moist muffins are packed with fiber and nutrition. Serve them warm with some whipped honey.

INGREDIENTS | YIELDS 18 MUFFINS

1 cup all-purpose flour

1 cup whole-wheat flour

2 tablespoons oat bran

2 tablespoons ground flaxseed

½ cup brown sugar

½ cup sugar

2 teaspoons cinnamon

¼ teaspoon nutmeg

1½ teaspoons baking powder

1 teaspoon baking soda

2 apples, peeled and chopped

1 cup grated carrots

½ cup applesauce

1 egg

1 egg white

¼ cup low-fat sour cream

¼ cup canola oil

2 teaspoons vanilla

1 cup dried cranberries

1 cup chopped walnuts

1. Preheat oven to 375°F. Line 18 muffin cups with paper liners and set aside. In a large bowl, combine all-purpose flour, whole-wheat flour, oat bran, flaxseed, brown sugar, sugar, cinnamon, nutmeg, baking powder, and baking soda and mix well.

2. In a medium bowl, combine apples, carrots, applesauce, egg, egg white, sour cream, canola oil, and vanilla, and beat to combine. Add to flour mixture and stir just until dry ingredients are moistened. Fold in cranberries and walnuts.

3. Fill prepared muffin cups three-quarters full. Bake for 15–25 minutes, or until muffins are golden-brown and a toothpick inserted in the center comes out clean. Remove from muffin cups and cool on a wire rack.

CALORIES: 210.22 | Fat: 8.48g | Saturated fat: 0.86g | Dietary fiber: 2.78g | Sodium: 116.29mg | Cholesterol: 13.06mg

Blueberry-Walnut Muffins

Blueberry muffins for breakfast are a great treat. Serve these warm from the oven.

INGREDIENTS | YIELDS 12 MUFFINS

1 cup buttermilk

1 egg

2 egg whites

6 tablespoons canola oil

½ cup sugar

⅛ teaspoon salt

1¼ cups plus 1 tablespoon all-purpose
flour

¾ cup whole-wheat flour

1 teaspoon baking powder

1 teaspoon baking soda

1 cup blueberries

½ cup chopped walnuts

2 tablespoons brown sugar

½ teaspoon cinnamon

Toss with Flour

It's best to toss fruit or nuts with a bit of flour before stirring into any batter. The flour helps hold these ingredients suspended in the batter, so they don't sink to the bottom as the bread bakes and rises in the oven. You need to use about 1 tablespoon of flour per cup of fruits or nuts.

1. Preheat oven to 400°F. Line 12 muffin cups with paper liners and set aside. In a large bowl, combine buttermilk, egg, egg whites, oil, sugar, and salt and mix well.

2. Stir in 1¼ cups all-purpose flour, whole-wheat flour, baking powder, and baking soda just until dry ingredients are moistened. In a small bowl, toss blueberries with 1 tablespoon flour. Stir into batter along with walnuts.

3. Fill prepared muffin cups ¾ full. In small bowl, combine 2 tablespoons brown sugar and cinnamon and sprinkle over muffins. Bake for 17–22 minutes or until golden-brown and set. Remove from muffin cups and cool on wire racks.

CALORIES: 230.36 | Fat: 10.80g | Saturated fat: 0.95g | Dietary fiber: 1.91g | Sodium: 197.52mg | Cholesterol: 18.44mg

Whole-Grain Corn Bread

Corn bread should be eaten hot from the oven. Instead of slathering it with butter, spread with whipped honey or top with Super-Spicy Salsa (Chapter 16).

INGREDIENTS | SERVES 9

¾ cup all-purpose flour

½ cup whole-wheat flour

¼ cup brown sugar

2 teaspoons baking powder

1 teaspoon baking soda

1 cup cornmeal

⅓ cup oat bran

1 egg

2 egg whites

¼ cup honey

1 cup buttermilk

¼ cup canola oil

1. Preheat oven to 400°F. Spray a 9" square pan with nonstick cooking spray containing flour, and set aside. In a large mixing bowl, combine all-purpose flour, whole-wheat flour, brown sugar, baking powder, baking soda, cornmeal, and oat bran and mix well.

2. In a small bowl, combine egg, egg whites, honey, buttermilk, and canola oil and beat to combine. Add to dry ingredients and stir just until mixed.

3. Spoon into prepared pan and smooth top. Bake for 25–35 minutes or until bread is golden-brown.

CALORIES: 252.79 | Fat: 7.58g | Saturated fat: 0.87g | Dietary fiber: 2.79g | Sodium: 272.96mg | Cholesterol: 24.59mg

Oat-Bran Date Muffins

*Dates contain lots of soluble fiber and are naturally sweet.
Keep some Medjool dates on hand for snacking.*

INGREDIENTS | YIELDS 12 MUFFINS

1¼ cups all-purpose flour

½ cup rolled oats

¼ cup oat bran

1½ teaspoons baking powder

1 teaspoon baking soda

⅓ cup brown sugar

1 egg

¼ cup canola oil

⅓ cup applesauce

1 teaspoon grated orange zest

1 cup finely chopped dates

½ cup chopped hazelnuts

1. Preheat oven to 350°F. Line 12 muffin cups with paper liners and set aside. In a large bowl, combine flour, oats, oat bran, baking powder, baking soda, and brown sugar, and mix well.

2. In a medium bowl, combine egg, canola oil, applesauce, and orange zest. Beat to combine. Add to dry ingredients and stir just until moistened. Fold in dates and hazelnuts.

3. Fill muffin cups two-thirds full. Bake for 25–35 minutes or until a toothpick inserted in the center comes out clean. Remove from muffin cups to wire racks to cool.

CALORIES: 232.40 | Fat: 8.66g | Saturated fat: 0.80g | Dietary fiber: 3.37g | Sodium: 159.46mg | Cholesterol: 17.63mg

Pumpkin Bread

This spicy and velvety bread has the best aroma while it's baking, and it tastes even better.

INGREDIENTS | YIELDS 1 LOAF; 12 SERVINGS

½ cup brown sugar

¼ cup plus 2 tablespoons sugar

¼ cup canola oil

1 egg

2 egg whites

2 teaspoons vanilla

1 cup canned solid-pack no-salt pumpkin

1¼ cups all-purpose flour

½ cup whole-wheat flour

1 teaspoon baking powder

½ teaspoon baking soda

1 teaspoon cinnamon, divided

¼ teaspoon nutmeg

¼ teaspoon cardamom

1. Preheat oven to 350°F. Spray a 9" × 5" loaf pan with nonstick cooking spray containing flour, and set aside.

2. In a large bowl, combine brown sugar, ¼ cup sugar, canola oil, egg, egg whites, and vanilla and beat until combined. Add pumpkin and beat until smooth.

3. Sift together all-purpose flour, whole-wheat flour, baking powder, baking soda, ½ teaspoon cinnamon, nutmeg, and cardamom. Add to pumpkin mixture and beat until smooth.

4. Spoon batter into prepared pan. In a small bowl combine 2 tablespoons sugar and ½ teaspoon cinnamon and mix well. Sprinkle over batter. Bake for 60–70 minutes or until bread is set and a toothpick inserted in the center comes out clean. Remove from pan and let cool on wire rack.

CALORIES: 178.02 | Fat: 5.63g | Saturated fat: 0.64g | Dietary fiber: 1.48g | Sodium: 108.61mg | Cholesterol: 35.25mg

Whole-Wheat Cinnamon Platters

These crisp and flat rolls are a perfect treat for a special occasion, like Christmas morning or Mother's Day.

INGREDIENTS | YIELDS 18 PLATTERS

1 cup whole-wheat flour

1 (¼-ounce) package instant-blend dry yeast

1¼ to 1¾ cups all-purpose flour, divided

¼ teaspoon salt

3 teaspoons cinnamon

⅛ teaspoon cardamom

2 tablespoons honey

¼ cup orange juice

1 tablespoon butter

½ cup water

1 egg

1 cup dried currants

1 cup sugar

1 cup finely chopped walnuts

1. In a large bowl, combine whole-wheat flour, yeast, ½ cup all-purpose flour, salt, 1 teaspoon cinnamon, and cardamom and mix well. In small saucepan, combine honey, orange juice, butter, and water; heat until very warm. Add to flour mixture and beat for 2 minutes.

2. Add egg and beat for 1 minute. Stir in enough remaining all-purpose flour to form a stiff batter. Stir in currants. Cover and let rise for 1 hour.

3. Stir down dough. Line cookie sheets with parchment paper or Silpat liners. On a plate, combine sugar, walnuts, and 2 teaspoons cinnamon and mix well. Drop dough by spoonfuls into the sugar mixture and toss to coat. Place on prepared cookie sheets and flatten to ⅛" thick circles.

4. Preheat oven to 400°F. Bake pastries for 13–16 minutes or until light golden-brown and caramelized. Let cool on cookie sheets for 3 minutes, then remove to wire rack to cool.

CALORIES: 189.56 | Fat: 5.30g | Saturated fat: 0.77g | Dietary fiber: 2.41g | Sodium: 42.47mg | Cholesterol: 13.44mg

Whole-Grain Oatmeal Bread

This hearty bread is delicious toasted and spread with whipped honey or jam.

INGREDIENTS | YIELDS 2 LOAVES; 32 SERVINGS

1 cup warm water

2 (¼-ounce) packages active dry yeast

¼ cup honey

1 cup skim milk

1 cup oatmeal

1 teaspoon salt

3 tablespoons canola oil

1 egg

1½ cups whole-wheat flour

½ cup medium rye flour

¼ cup ground flaxseed

3 to 4 cups bread flour

2 tablespoons butter, melted

Rolls or Bread?

You can make rolls out of any yeast bread mixture. Just divide the dough into 2" balls and roll between your hands to smooth. Place on greased cookie sheets about 4" apart. Cover and let rise for 30–40 minutes. Then bake at 375°F for 15–25 minutes until deep golden-brown. Let cool on wire racks. Freeze if not using within 1 day.

1. In a small bowl, combine water and yeast; let stand until bubbly, about 5 minutes. Meanwhile, in medium saucepan combine honey, milk, oatmeal, salt, and canola oil. Heat just until very warm (about 120°F). Remove from heat and beat in egg. Combine in large bowl with whole-wheat flour, rye flour, flaxseed, and 1 cup bread flour. Add yeast mixture and beat for 1 minute. Cover and let rise for 30 minutes.

2. Gradually stir in enough remaining bread flour to make a firm dough. Turn onto floured surface and knead until dough is elastic, about 10 minutes. Place in greased bowl, turning to grease top. Cover and let rise for 1 hour. Punch down dough, divide in half, and form into loaves. Place in greased 9" × 5" loaf pans, cover, and let rise for 30 minutes.

3. Bake in a preheated 350°F oven for 25–30 minutes or until golden-brown. Brush with butter, then remove to wire racks to cool.

CALORIES: 136.74 | Fat: 3.46g | Saturated fat: 0.77g | Dietary fiber: 2.25g | Sodium: 85.39mg | Cholesterol: 8.67mg

Oat Bran Dinner Rolls

These excellent rolls are light yet hearty, with a wonderful flavor and a bit of crunch.

INGREDIENTS | **YIELDS 30 ROLLS**

1½ cups water

¾ cup quick-cooking oats

½ cup plus 2 tablespoons oat bran

¼ cup brown sugar

2 tablespoons butter or plant sterol margarine

1 cup buttermilk

2 ¼-ounce packages active dry yeast

2 to 3 cups all-purpose flour, divided

1½ cups whole-wheat flour

½ teaspoon salt

2 tablespoons honey

1 egg white, beaten

1. In a medium saucepan, bring water to a boil over high heat. Add oats, ½ cup oat bran, brown sugar, and butter and stir until butter melts. Remove from heat and let cool to lukewarm.

2. Meanwhile, in a microwave-safe glass cup, place buttermilk. Microwave on medium for 1 minute or until lukewarm (about 110°F). Sprinkle yeast over milk; stir and let stand for 10 minutes.

3. In a large mixing bowl, combine 1 cup all-purpose flour, whole-wheat flour, and salt. Add honey, cooled oatmeal mixture, and softened yeast mixture and beat until smooth. Gradually add enough remaining all-purpose flour to form a soft dough.

4. Turn onto lightly floured board and knead until smooth and elastic, about 5–7 minutes. Place in greased bowl, turning to grease top. Cover and let rise for 1 hour or until dough doubles.

5. Punch down dough and divide into thirds. Divide each third into 10 pieces. Roll balls between your hands to smooth. Place balls into two 9" round cake pans. Brush with egg white and sprinkle with 2 tablespoons oat bran. Cover and let rise until doubled, about 45 minutes.

6. Preheat oven to 375°F. Bake rolls for 15–25 minutes or until firm to the touch and golden-brown. Remove from pans and cool on wire racks.

CALORIES: 100.84 | Fat: 1.48g | Saturated fat: 0.64g | Dietary fiber: 1.83g | Sodium: 54.45mg | Cholesterol: 2.36mg

Honey-Wheat Sesame Bread

Sesame seeds add not only flavor and crunch to these delicious loaves but fiber and healthy monounsaturated fat as well.

INGREDIENTS | YIELDS 2 LOAVES; 32 SERVINGS

1 cup milk

1 cup water

½ cup honey

3 tablespoons butter

¼ teaspoon salt

1 egg

2 cups whole-wheat flour

2 (¼-ounce) packages instant-blend dry yeast

½ cup sesame seeds

3 to 4 cups all-purpose flour

Unsalted butter, as needed

1 egg white

2 tablespoons sesame seeds

1. In a medium saucepan, combine milk, water, honey, butter, and salt. Heat over medium heat until butter melts. Remove from heat and let stand for 30 minutes or until just lukewarm. Beat in egg.

2. Meanwhile, in a large bowl combine whole-wheat flour, instant-blend yeast, and ½ cup sesame seeds. Add milk mixture and beat for 1 minute. Then gradually stir in enough all-purpose flour to make a firm dough.

3. Turn out onto floured surface and knead, adding additional flour if necessary, until dough is elastic. Place in greased bowl, turning to grease top; cover and let rise until doubled, about 1 hour.

4. Grease two 9" × 5" loaf pans with unsalted butter and set aside. Punch down dough and divide into two parts. On floured surface, roll or pat to 7" × 12" rectangle. Roll up tightly, starting with 7" side. Place in prepared pans. Brush with egg white and sprinkle each with 1 tablespoon sesame seeds.

5. Cover with towel, and let rise until doubled, about 30 minutes. Preheat oven to 350°F. Bake loaves for 35–45 minutes or until golden-brown. Turn onto a wire rack to cool completely.

CALORIES: 131.38 | Fat: 3.02g | Saturated fat: 1.03g | Dietary fiber: 1.77g | Sodium: 34.51mg | Cholesterol: 9.85mg

Raisin-Cinnamon Oatmeal Bread

Batter breads are really simple to make because they require less of your time.

INGREDIENTS | YIELDS 2 LOAVES; 32 SERVINGS

2 ¼-ounce packages active dry yeast

½ cup warm water

1¼ cups skim milk

¼ cup brown sugar

¼ cup honey

1 egg

2 egg whites

⅓ cup oat bran

1¼ cups oatmeal

3½ to 4½ cups all-purpose flour

½ teaspoon salt

2 teaspoons cinnamon

2 cups raisins

2 tablespoons butter, melted

Batter Breads

Batter breads are just breads with less flour, so instead of forming a dough they make a stiff batter that becomes difficult to stir. Because the bread isn't kneaded and there is more liquid, the texture of the bread comes out coarser. These breads are quicker to make and are less intimidating to beginning cooks.

1. In a large bowl, combine yeast and warm water; let stand for 10 minutes. In a small saucepan, combine milk, brown sugar, and honey; heat over low heat until warm. Add to yeast along with egg and egg whites; beat until combined.

2. Add oat bran, oatmeal, and 1 cup all-purpose flour and beat for 1 minute. Let stand, covered, for 30 minutes. Then stir in salt, cinnamon, raisins, and enough all-purpose flour to form a stiff batter; beat for 2 minutes.

3. Spray two 9" × 5" loaf pans with nonstick cooking spray. Divide batter among the pans, smoothing the top. Cover and let rise for 45 minutes until batter is doubled.

4. Preheat oven to 375°F. Bake bread for 30–40 minutes or until bread is firm and golden-brown. Remove from pans, brush tops with melted butter, and let cool on wire racks.

CALORIES: 138.98 | Fat: 1.60g | Saturated fat: 0.63g | Dietary fiber: 1.65g | Sodium: 54.50mg | Cholesterol: 8.71g

Sunflower Rye Bread

Forming the dough into a round and baking it on a cookie sheet makes a rustic loaf that is crustier than bread baked in a loaf pan.

INGREDIENTS | YIELDS 1 LOAF; 16 SERVINGS

½ cup lukewarm water

1 (¼-ounce) package active dry yeast

⅔ cup skim milk

¼ cup honey

½ teaspoon salt

2 tablespoons canola oil

1 egg, beaten, divided

1 cup medium rye flour

½ cup whole-wheat flour

2 to 3 cups bread flour

1 cup hulled unsalted sunflower seeds

1. In a small bowl combine water and yeast and let stand until bubbly, about 5 minutes. In a microwave-safe glass bowl, combine milk, honey, salt, and canola oil and heat on 30 percent power until warm, about 30–40 seconds. Pour milk mixture into a large bowl.

2. Remove 1 tablespoon egg and refrigerate for glaze. Add remaining egg to milk mixture along with yeast mixture and rye flour; beat for 1 minute. Add whole-wheat flour and 1 cup bread flour; beat for 1 minute.

3. Gradually stir in enough remaining bread flour to form a firm dough. On a lightly floured surface, knead in sunflower seeds. Knead bread until smooth and elastic, about 10 minutes. Place in greased bowl, turning to grease top. Cover and let rise for 1 hour.

4. Punch down dough and let rest for 10 minutes. Spray a cookie sheet with nonstick cooking spray. On a floured surface, shape dough into an 8" round. Place on a prepared cookie sheet. Brush with reserved egg, cover, and let rise for 30 minutes. Bake for 35–45 minutes or until dark golden-brown. Let cool on a wire rack.

CALORIES: 199.73 | Fat: 6.57g | Saturated fat: 0.73g | Dietary fiber: 2.89g | Sodium: 83.83mg | Cholesterol: 13.42mg

Whole-Grain Pizza Crust

Make a couple of batches of this crust, prebake, and store in the freezer to make your own homemade pizzas in a flash.

INGREDIENTS | YIELDS 2 CRUSTS; 12 SERVINGS

1 cup warm water

2 ¼-ounce packages active dry yeast

½ cup skim milk

2 tablespoons honey

2 tablespoons olive oil

½ teaspoon salt

1½ cups whole-wheat flour

1 cup cornmeal, plus more as needed

1½ to 2½ cups bread flour

Freezing Pizza Dough

To freeze pizza dough, bake it for 10 minutes until the crust is set but not browned. Let cool completely, then place in heavy-duty food storage freezer bags, seal, label, and freeze for up to 3 months. To use, you can top the crust right from the freezer and bake as recipe directs, adding 5–10 minutes to the baking time.

1. In a large bowl, combine water and yeast; let stand for 10 minutes until bubbly. Add milk, honey, olive oil, and salt and mix well. Stir in whole-wheat flour, 1 cup cornmeal, and ½ cup bread flour; beat for 1 minute.

2. Stir in enough bread flour to make a firm dough. Turn onto floured surface and knead for 10 minutes. Place dough in greased bowl, turning to grease top. Cover and let rise for 1 hour.

3. Turn dough onto a floured work surface and let rest for 10 minutes. Spray two 12" round pizza pans with nonstick cooking spray and sprinkle with some cornmeal. Divide dough in half and roll to 12" circles; place on pizza pans; press to edges if necessary. Let stand for 10 minutes.

4. Preheat oven to 400°F. Bake crusts for 10 minutes or until set. Remove from oven, add toppings, return to oven, and bake as the pizza recipe directs.

CALORIES: 213.01 | Fat: 3.17g | Saturated fat: 0.46g | Dietary fiber: 3.48g | Sodium: 104.52mg | Cholesterol: 0.20mg

Light Whole-Grain Bread

This hearty, crunchy loaf is packed full of flavor, nutrition, and fiber.

INGREDIENTS | YIELDS 2 LOAVES; 32 SERVINGS

1 cup lukewarm water
2 (¼-ounce) packages active dry yeast
1½ cups buttermilk
½ cup orange juice
½ teaspoon salt
⅓ cup honey
3 tablespoons canola oil
1 egg
2 cups whole-wheat flour
½ cup oat bran
½ cup cracked wheat
3½ to 4½ cups bread flour
½ teaspoon baking soda
Unsalted butter, as needed
2 tablespoons melted butter

1. In a large bowl, combine water and yeast; mix well and let stand for 10 minutes. Add buttermilk, orange juice, salt, honey, oil, and egg and beat well. Add 1 cup whole-wheat flour, oat bran, cracked wheat, 1 cup bread flour, and baking soda; beat for 1 minute. Let bread stand for 30 minutes.

2. Gradually add enough remaining whole-wheat flour and bread flour to form a firm dough. Turn onto a floured surface and knead for 10 minutes. Place dough in greased bowl, turning to grease top. Cover and let rise for 1 hour.

3. Turn dough onto a floured work surface and let rest for 10 minutes. Grease two 9" × 5" loaf pans with unsalted butter and set aside. Punch down dough and divide into two parts. On a floured surface, roll or pat to 7" × 12" rectangle. Roll up tightly, starting with the 7" side. Place in prepared pans.

4. Cover with a towel, and let rise until doubled, about 30 minutes. Preheat oven to 350°F. Bake loaves for 35–45 minutes or until golden-brown. Brush each loaf with butter, then turn onto wire rack to cool completely.

CALORIES: 137.87 | Fat: 2.75g | Saturated fat: 0.74g | Dietary fiber: 2.16g | Sodium: 76.58mg | Cholesterol: 8.98mg

Whole-Grain Ciabatta

Ciabatta means "slipper" in Italian. The loaves are fairly flat and oblong, with large air holes and a nice crust.

INGREDIENTS | YIELDS 2 LOAVES; 8 SERVINGS

1 cup lukewarm water

1¼-ounce package active dry yeast

⅓ cup milk

2 tablespoons olive oil

¾ cup whole-wheat flour

½ cup oat bran

2 to 2½ cups bread flour

½ teaspoon salt

2 tablespoons cornmeal

Creating Steam When Baking Bread

Adding steam to the oven when baking bread makes a crisper, thicker crust. There are several ways to do this. You can place a pan with some water in it on the rack below the bread. You can also spritz the loaves with water a few times while the bread is baking. The steam helps keep the bread softer longer, so the crust develops more slowly.

1. In a large bowl, combine water and yeast; stir and let stand for 10 minutes. When yeast is bubbly, add milk, olive oil, whole-wheat flour, oat bran, ½ cup bread flour, and salt and beat for 2 minutes. Cover and let stand at room temperature for 1 hour.

2. Add enough remaining bread flour to make a soft dough; beat for 1 minute. Cover bowl and let rise for 1 hour.

3. Remove dough to lightly floured surface (dough will be soft and sticky). Grease two 4" × 10" shapes on a large cookie sheet and sprinkle with cornmeal. Divide dough in half and shape into two 3" × 9" rectangles on the greased areas of the cookie sheet. Let rise for 30 minutes.

4. Preheat oven to 400°F. Place a 9" pan filled with ½" of water on the bottom rack. Bake bread on the middle rack for 20–30 minutes or until loaves are light golden-brown and sound hollow when tapped with fingers. Cool on a wire rack.

CALORIES: 212.26 | Fat: 4.62g | Saturated fat: 0.68g | Dietary fiber: 3.28g | Sodium: 152.68mg | Cholesterol: 0.20mg

Three-Grain French Bread

Yogurt and orange juice add a bit of sourdough texture and flavor to this easy and delicious loaf.

INGREDIENTS | YIELDS 2 LOAVES; 16 SERVINGS

¾ cup warm water

2 ¼-ounce packages active dry yeast

1 tablespoon sugar

¼ cup orange juice

1 cup plain yogurt

2 tablespoons lemon juice

1 egg

⅓ cup oat bran

½ teaspoon salt

1½ cups whole-wheat flour

3 to 3½ cups bread flour

1 tablespoon cornmeal

Storing French Bread

Homemade French bread will not last very long after it's baked. Within two days of baking the bread, slice it into 1" slices and flash freeze on a cookie sheet. When the bread is frozen, pack into hard-sided containers, label, seal, and freeze up to 3 months. To use, spread with olive oil and toast right out of the freezer.

1. In a large bowl, combine water, yeast, and sugar; stir and let stand for 10 minutes. Add orange juice, yogurt, lemon juice, and egg and beat for 1 minute. Add oat bran, salt, whole-wheat flour, and 1 cup bread flour and beat. Cover for 1 hour.

2. Gradually add enough remaining bread flour to form a firm dough. Turn onto a floured surface and knead for 10 minutes until smooth and elastic. Place in a greased bowl, turning to grease top. Cover and let rise for 1 hour.

3. Punch down dough and let rest for 10 minutes. With nonstick cooking spray, spray two 14" × 4" rectangles on a cookie sheet and sprinkle with cornmeal. Divide dough in half and roll each half to a 14" × 6" rectangle. Roll up tightly, starting at the longer side. Pinch edges and ends to seal and place, seam side down, onto prepared cookie sheet.

4. Cover and let rise for 30 minutes, or until doubled. Preheat oven to 375°F. Slash bread in shallow cuts several times, cutting across the loaves, using a sharp knife. Bake for 30–40 minutes or until loaves are golden-brown and sound hollow when tapped with fingers. Let cool on a wire rack.

CALORIES: 158.22 | Fat: 1.61g | Saturated fat: 0.53g | Dietary fiber: 2.52g | Sodium: 85.22mg | Cholesterol: 15.06mg

Savory French Toast

French toast doesn't have to be sweet! This version is delicious topped with spicy tomato sauce.

INGREDIENTS | SERVES 4–6

1 tablespoon olive oil

1 tablespoon butter

1 onion, chopped

4 1"-thick slices Light Whole-Grain Bread (see recipe in this chapter)

1 cup shredded Jarlsberg cheese

1 egg

1 egg white

⅓ cup buttermilk

1 teaspoon dried thyme leaves

½ teaspoon hot sauce

1 cup Spaghetti Sauce (Chapter 18)

1. In a large saucepan, combine olive oil and butter over medium heat. Add onion; cook and stir until tender, about 5 minutes. Continue cooking until onion begins to turn golden, about 5–8 minutes longer. Remove onion from pan and place in a small bowl. Remove pan from heat.

2. Let onion cool for 15 minutes. Meanwhile, cut a pocket in the center of each slice of bread. Add Jarlsberg to the onion mixture and mix. Stuff this into the bread pockets.

3. In a shallow bowl, combine egg, egg whites, buttermilk, thyme, and hot sauce, and beat well. Dip stuffed bread into egg mixture, turning to coat.

4. Return saucepan to heat. Sauté the stuffed bread, turning once, about 4–5 minutes on each side until golden-brown. Serve with warmed Spaghetti Sauce.

CALORIES: 342.51 | Fat: 14.56g | Saturated fat: 6.14g | Dietary fiber: 3.98g | Sodium: 198.74mg | Cholesterol: 65.18mg

Caesar Dressing

This creamy and flavorful dressing is usually made with raw eggs.
Using low-fat mayonnaise instead is a better choice for food-safety reasons.

INGREDIENTS | **YIELDS 1 CUP; SERVING SIZE 2 TABLESPOONS**

1 garlic clove, minced

1 anchovy fillet

½ cup low-fat mayonnaise

¼ cup plain yogurt

2 tablespoons lemon juice

¼ cup olive oil

¼ teaspoon pepper

⅓ cup grated Parmesan cheese

Combine garlic, anchovy, mayonnaise, yogurt, and lemon juice in blender or food processor. Blend or process until smooth. Stream in olive oil while blending or processing, until smooth. Add pepper and Parmesan and mix well; cover and refrigerate for up to 4 days.

CALORIES: 152.79 | Fat: 14.82g | Saturated fat: 2.80g | Dietary fiber: 0.02g | Sodium: 137.29mg | Cholesterol: 4.55mg

Balsamic Vinaigrette

This is an incredibly versatile dressing. You can add all sorts of different herbs to it;
thyme and rosemary would be delicious.

INGREDIENTS | **SERVES 9; SERVING SIZE 2 TABLESPOONS**

⅔ cup extra-virgin olive oil

⅓ cup aged balsamic vinegar

1 teaspoon Worcestershire sauce

2 cloves garlic, minced

1 tablespoon lemon juice

1 tablespoon honey

¼ teaspoon salt

⅛ teaspoon white pepper

Whisk all ingredients together. Cover and store in refrigerator for up to 3 days. Drizzle over salad greens or use as called for in recipes.

CALORIES: 151.96 | Fat: 16.00g | Saturated fat: 2.21g | Dietary fiber: 0.03g | Sodium: 71.49mg | Cholesterol: 0.0mg

Lite Creamy Cheesecake

The secret to this cheesecake is to make sure that the cottage cheese is completely smooth before proceeding with the recipe.

INGREDIENTS | SERVES 12

1½ cups crushed gingersnap crumbs

⅓ cup finely chopped walnuts

2 tablespoons butter or margarine, melted

2 tablespoons plus ¼ cup orange juice

1½ cups nonfat cottage cheese

1 cup sugar

2 tablespoons lemon juice

1 8-ounce package light cream cheese, softened

1 3-ounce package nonfat cream cheese, softened

1 cup nonfat sour cream

1 egg

3 egg whites

¼ cup cornstarch

1 tablespoon vanilla

1. Preheat oven to 350°F. In a medium bowl, combine gingersnap crumbs, walnuts, butter, and 2 tablespoons orange juice; mix until even. Press into bottom and up the sides of a 9" springform pan; set aside in refrigerator.

2. In a blender or food processor, combine cottage cheese, sugar, ¼ cup orange juice, and lemon juice; blend or process until very smooth. Scrape down sides and blend or process again.

3. In a large mixing bowl, combine both packages of cream cheese and beat until smooth. Add sour cream; beat again until smooth. Add egg and beat well, then add cottage cheese mixture and beat well. Stir in egg whites, cornstarch, and vanilla and beat until smooth.

4. Pour cheese mixture onto gingersnap crust. Bake for 50–60 minutes or until cheesecake is set around edges but still soft in center. Remove from oven and place on a wire rack; let cool for 1 hour. Cover and refrigerate until cold, at least 4 hours.

CALORIES: 254.77 | Fat: 9.11g | Saturated fat: 4.07g | Dietary fiber: 0.49g | Sodium: 206.98mg | Cholesterol: 37.05mg

Silken Chocolate Mousse

This velvety-smooth and rich mousse has the best texture.
Top it with some fresh raspberries for the perfect finish.

INGREDIENTS | SERVES 6

2 1-ounce squares unsweetened chocolate

2 tablespoons butter

½ cup sugar

1 teaspoon vanilla

½ cup satin or silken soft tofu

1 cup chocolate frozen yogurt

1 cup frozen nondairy whipped topping, thawed

Silken Tofu

Make sure that you use silken tofu in this or any other mousse or pudding recipe. Do not use the block type that floats in water. Silken tofu may be packaged in aseptic packaging and stocked on the grocery shelves, not the dairy aisle. All tofu is made of the same ingredients; it's processed differently to make the different types.

1. Chop chocolate and place in a small microwave-safe bowl with the butter. Microwave on medium for 2–4 minutes, stirring twice during cooking time, until chocolate is melted and mixture is smooth. Stir in sugar until sugar dissolves.

2. In a blender or food processor, place chocolate mixture and add vanilla and tofu. Blend or process until smooth. If necessary, let cool for 10–15 minutes or until lukewarm.

3. Then add the frozen yogurt and blend or process until smooth. Finally, add the whipped topping and blend or process until just mixed. Spoon into serving glasses, cover, and chill for 4–6 hours before serving.

CALORIES: 219.73 | Fat: 12.12g | Saturated fat: 7.86g | Dietary fiber: 2.13g | Sodium: 78.14mg | Cholesterol: 11.62mg

Whole-Wheat Chocolate Chip Cookies

Fill your cookie jar with these excellent cookies!
They're high in fiber yet studded with delicious dark-chocolate nuggets.

INGREDIENTS | YIELDS 48 COOKIES

¼ cup butter or plant sterol margarine, softened

1½ cups brown sugar

½ cup applesauce

1 tablespoon vanilla

1 egg

2 egg whites

2½ cups whole-wheat pastry flour

½ cup ground oatmeal

1 teaspoon baking soda

¼ teaspoon salt

2 cups special dark chocolate chips

1 cup chopped hazelnuts

1. Preheat oven to 375°F. Line cookie sheets with parchment paper or Silpat silicone liners and set aside.

2. In large bowl, combine butter, brown sugar, and applesauce and beat well until smooth. Add vanilla, egg, and egg whites and beat until combined.

3. Add flour, oatmeal, baking soda, and salt and mix until a dough forms. Fold in chocolate chips and hazelnuts.

4. Drop dough by rounded teaspoons onto prepared cookie sheets. Bake for 7–10 minutes or until cookies are light golden-brown and set. Let cool for 5 minutes before removing from cookie sheet to a wire rack to cool.

CALORIES: 114.86 | Fat: 4.89g | Saturated fat: 2.04g | Dietary fiber: 1.62g | Sodium: 26.49mg | Cholesterol: 6.95mg

Whole-Wheat Pastry Flour

Whole-wheat pastry flour isn't the same as whole-wheat flour; it's slightly lighter and finer for baking. You can find it in specialty stores and online. You can substitute plain whole-wheat flour if you can't find the pastry flour, but use 2 tablespoons less per cup. Plain flour is denser, with a stronger flavor.

Oatmeal Brownies

Ground oatmeal, prune purée, and finely chopped dates add great chewy texture (and fiber) to these easy brownies.

INGREDIENTS | YIELDS 16 BROWNIES

¼ cup prune purée

¼ cup finely chopped dates

½ cup all-purpose flour

½ cup ground oatmeal

½ cup cocoa powder

½ teaspoon baking soda

½ cup brown sugar

¼ cup sugar

1 egg

1 egg white

¼ cup chocolate yogurt

2 teaspoons vanilla

2 tablespoons butter or plant sterol margarine, melted

½ cup dark chocolate chips

1. Preheat oven to 350°F. Spray an 8" square baking pan with nonstick cooking spray containing flour and set aside.

2. In a small bowl, combine prune purée and dates; mix well and set aside. In a large bowl, combine flour, oatmeal, cocoa, baking soda, brown sugar, and sugar and mix well.

3. Add egg, egg white, yogurt, vanilla, and butter to prune mixture and mix well. Add to flour mixture and stir just until blended. Spoon into prepared pan and smooth top. Bake for 22–30 minutes or until edges are set but the center is still slightly soft. Remove from oven and place on wire rack.

4. In a microwave-safe bowl, place chocolate chips. Microwave on 50 percent power for 1 minute, then remove and stir. Microwave for 30 seconds longer, then stir. If necessary, repeat microwave process until chips are melted. Pour over warm brownies and gently spread to cover. Let cool completely and cut into bars.

CALORIES: 153.83 | Fat: 4.88g | Saturated fat: 2.63g | Dietary fiber: 2.54g | Sodium: 63.58mg | Cholesterol: 17.39mg

Resources

Cholesterol Resources

American Heart Association
www.americanheart.org/cholesterol

Harvard Cholesterol Nutrition Guide
www.hsph.harvard.edu/nutritionsource/what-should-you-eat/fats-and-cholesterol

National Cholesterol Education Program
www.nhlbi.nih.gov/about/ncep

NIH ATP3 Cholesterol Guidelines
www.nhlbi.nih.gov/guidelines/cholesterol

WebMD Cholesterol Management Center
www.webmd.com/cholesterol-management

Cardiovascular Disease Resources

American Diabetes Association
www.diabetes.org

American Heart Association
www.americanheart.org

American Lung Association
www.lungusa.org

Cardiovascular Risk-Assessment Calculator
http://hp2010.nhlbihin.net/atpiii/calculator.asp

Stanford Prevention Resource Center, Stanford University School of Medicine
http://prevention.stanford.edu

Health Organization Resources

American Red Cross
www.redcross.org

Centers for Disease Control and Prevention (CDC)
www.cdc.gov

National Heart, Lung, and Blood Institute
www.nhlbi.nih.gov

National Institute of Diabetes and Digestive and Kidney Diseases (NIDDK)
www.niddk.nih.gov

National Institutes of Health
www.nih.gov

U.S. Department of Agriculture (USDA)
www.usda.gov

U.S. Department of Health and Human Services
www.dhhs.gov

U.S. Food and Drug Administration (FDA)
www.fda.gov

Smoking Cessation Resources

American Cancer Society
www.cancer.org/docroot/PED/content/PED_10_13X_Guide_for_Quitting_Smoking.asp

CDC Office on Smoking and Health
www.cdc.gov/tobacco

Smokefree.gov
http://smokefree.gov

Stop Smoking Foundation
www.stopsmoking.net

Food and Nutrition Resources

American Dietetic Association
www.eatright.org

Food and Nutrition Information Center
www.nal.usda.gov/fnic

Organic Food Resources

Horizon Organic Dairy
www.horizonorganic.com

The National Directory of Farmers Markets
www.ams.usda.gov/AMSv1.0/FarmersMarkets

Organic.org
http://organic.org

Organicfood.net
http://organicfood.net

Organic Trade Association
www.ota.com

USDA Agricultural Marketing Service
www.ams.usda.gov

Natural Food Chains

Trader Joe's
www.traderjoes.com

Whole Foods Market, Inc.
www.wholefoods.com

Obesity Resources

Centers For Disease Control and Prevention Obesity
www.cdc.gov/obesity

The Obesity Society
www.obesity.org

Weight-Control Information Network
www.niddk.nih.gov/health/nutrit/pubs/health.htm

World Health Organization Obesity
www.who.int/topics/obesity/en

Exercise Resources

Aerobics and Fitness Association of America (AFAA)
www.afaa.com

American College of Sports Medicine
www.acsm.org

American Council on Exercise
www.acefitness.org

American Senior Fitness Association
www.seniorfitness.net

Aquatic Exercise Association (AEA)
www.aeawave.com

Disabled Sports Organizations
www.dsusa.org

International Council for Active Aging
www.icaa.cc

Medical Fitness Association (MFA)
www.medicalfitness.org

The National Center on Physical Activity and Disability-Department of Disability and Human Development University of Illinois at Chicago
www.ncpad.org

National Strength and Conditioning Association
http://nsca-lift.org

President's Council on Physical Fitness and Sports
www.fitness.gov

YMCA of the USA
www.ymca.net

Stress and Wellness Resources

American Institute of Stress
www.stress.org

Learning Meditation
www.learningmeditation.com

Mayo Clinic Relaxation Techniques
www.mayoclinic.com/health/relaxation-technique/SR00007

The Meditation Society of America
www.meditationsociety.com

WebMD Stress Management Health Center
www.webmd.com/balance/stress-management/default.htm

Calculating Your Body Mass Index

The body mass index (BMI) is a measure that reduces the relationship between weight and height to one number. When you compare your BMI value to charted ranges, you get an approximation of body fatness, rather than a precise measure. The figure is not equal to a measurement of body-fat percentage.

The value of knowing your BMI is that it provides a rough estimate of whether your body size indicates a need to manage your weight more effectively.

To find your BMI, use the formula below, or check the Body Mass Index Chart for an approximate value. To understand what your BMI means, check the BMI categories for men and women. Overweight is defined as a BMI of 25 to 29.9; obesity is defined as a BMI equal to or more than 30. These numbers may not apply to pregnant women or muscular athletes.

Calculate Your BMI

The BMI was created using the metric system. To calculate your BMI, you can take your weight in kilograms and divide it by the square (a number multiplied by itself) of your height in meters. If you are more likely using pounds and inches, follow this simple three-step method:

Multiply your weight by 703.

Divide the result by your height.

Divide the result again by your height to get your BMI.

For example: If you are five foot seven (or 67 inches tall) and weigh 170 pounds, you would do the following:

Multiply 170×703 to get 119,510.

Divide 119,510 by 67 to get 1,785.

Divide 1,785 by 67 to get 26.6.

In this example, the BMI is 26.6; this BMI falls in the overweight category.

Body Mass Index Chart

For a less precise answer without the math, here is a chart for men and women that gives the body mass index (BMI) for various heights (in inches) and weights (in pounds, with underwear but no shoes). Find your height, read across the row to your weight, then read up the column to find your approximate BMI score.

The Body Mass Index Chart	21	22	23	24	25	26	27	28	29	30	31
4'10"	100	105	110	115	119	124	129	134	138	143	148
5'0"	107	112	118	123	128	133	138	143	148	153	158
5'1"	111	116	122	127	132	137	143	148	153	158	164
5'3"	118	124	130	135	141	146	152	158	163	169	175
5'5"	126	132	138	144	150	156	162	168	174	180	186
5'7"	134	140	146	153	159	166	172	178	185	191	198
5'9"	142	149	155	162	169	176	182	189	196	203	209
6'0"	150	157	165	172	179	186	193	200	208	215	222
6'1"	159	166	174	182	189	197	204	212	219	227	235
6'3"	168	176	184	192	200	208	216	224	232	240	248

What Does Your BMI Mean?

BMI ranges from 18.5 to 24.9.
Normal weight: Good for you! Try not to gain weight.

BMI ranges from 25 to 29.9.
Overweight: Try not to gain weight, especially if your waist measurement is high. You need to manage your weight if you have two or more risk factors for heart disease and are overweight, or have a high waist measurement.

BMI is 30 or greater.
Obese: You need to manage your weight. Lose weight slowly—about half a pound to two pounds a week. See your doctor or a registered dietitian if you need help.

Source: *Clinical Guidelines on the Identification, Evaluation, and Treatment of Overweight and Obesity in Adults*; National Heart, Lung, and Blood Institute, in cooperation with the National Institute of Diabetes and Digestive and Kidney Diseases, National Institutes of Health, June 1998.

Recipe Index

General Index

We Have EVERYTHING® on Anything!

With more than 19 million copies sold, the Everything® series has become one of America's favorite resources for solving problems, learning new skills, and organizing lives. Our brand is not only recognizable—it's also welcomed.

The series is a hand-in-hand partner for people who are ready to tackle new subjects—like you!

For more information on the Everything® series, please visit *www.adamsmedia.com*

The Everything® list spans a wide range of subjects, with more than 500 titles covering 25 different categories:

Business	History	Reference
Careers	Home Improvement	Religion
Children's Storybooks	Everything Kids	Self-Help
Computers	Languages	Sports & Fitness
Cooking	Music	Travel
Crafts and Hobbies	New Age	Wedding
Education/Schools	Parenting	Writing
Games and Puzzles	Personal Finance	
Health	Pets	